The Other Midlife Crisis

Arthritis and All Those Aches and Pains

D1291106

Michael R. Wilson, M.D.
Orthopedic Surgeon

Whiskey Hollow Press • New Orleans, LA
(504) 861-2188 • Fax (504) 861-1657
Printed by Garrity Printing

Cartoons on cover, back and
Chapter 1: The Syndromes by Walt Handelsman

Cover design by Upside Design: info@upsidedesign.net
Marketing and promotion by Rebecca O'Meara,
rebeccaomeara@aol.com.

Acknowledgements

You don't write a 350-page book without a lot of help. For me this whole project began as a chapter (The Syndromes) I wrote for a book that my wife, Dr. Kathy Wilson was writing on midlife medicine. Both books have morphed over the last two years, but our 30-year marriage and collaboration has remained the driving force behind getting these ideas into print.

I'd like to thank Walt Handelsman, who penned the terrific cartoons on the book cover and in the first chapter. He shared my vision of how funny boomers can be and put it on paper in the way only a Pulitzer Prize winning cartoonist can.

In the end, I owe the most to all my teachers, from the outstanding public school system in Iowa City, to the University of Iowa College of Medicine and the Mayo Clinic Department of Orthopaedics. But for any doctor the greatest teacher of all is his patients. As we say in surgery, "Experience is something that you gain, just after you needed it."

Disclaimer

This book is one orthopedic surgeon's very personal approach to the classification and treatment of the common musculoskeletal problems of midlife. It is intentionally opinionated and as such, presents my philosophy, developed over many years of treating patients. As there is often no one best treatment for many conditions, I do not present my view as the only view, or my way of treating patients as the only treatment. Please don't hold your doctor to my views. In a field as diverse and as dynamic as orthopedics, there will always be controversy, regional preferences and rapid developments.

A note on the spelling of "Orthopaedics": my certificate from the American Board of Orthopaedic Surgery spells the name of our specialty the old-fashioned way—with an "a" followed by an "e." So do all of our organizations. Unfortunately, every spell-checker, most magazines and newspapers and even Dorland's Medical Dictionary use the simpler "Orthopedics", without the fancy Greek diphthong, "ae." I chose the simple "e" spelling because I feel like we're fighting a losing battle here and currently only orthopods spell it the old way. I got tired of fighting the spell-checkers and editors.

In most cases the stories I've told are amalgams, composites of many patients. If you think you recognize yourself, you're wrong, except in those few cases where a patient has kindly consented to let me use his or her name and story.

Although I believe this information to be true and hope you find it helpful, I am not prescribing what any individual should do. The contents of the book are my professional opinion and I do not pretend to speak for other doctors. I do not intend this book as a standard of care reference. It is meant to teach, not to set some standard.

If you are an orthopedic surgeon and you disagree with anything I've said, go write your own book!

The Other Midlife Crisis

Table of Contents

Introduction

I first heard the line, "She was rode hard and put up wet" from Ronald Reagan. I can't even recall the context, but the Gipper was certainly a guy who could turn a phrase that would just epoxy onto your brain. That expression became a summary of the way I see my own generation, the baby boomers. You see, I'm an orthopedic surgeon and I have earned the privilege of treating the aching and the injured, the lucky and the lame—-those poor souls whose lives have tested the laws of physics and lost. I make my living at the fringes of the Law of Entropy, that immutable principle that all systems tend toward disorder. I'm the guy who's supposed to re-order things. I straighten what goes crooked, relocate what dislocates, replace what wears out and generally fix what's broken.

After 28 years as an orthopedist, I've noticed that the musculoskeletal problems of boomers tend to fall into certain categories, what I call "The Syndromes." It is these syndromes that separate us from all the other age groups that I treat. Old folks have their problems, children have their problems, but in midlife, we have a unique set of musculoskeletal complaints that I think can only be appreciated if you understand what's driving us. Make no mistake about it; we are the driven generation. We are driven to succeed and driven to exceed. Sometimes we push way too hard, and that's where I come in.

In this book I'll first introduce you to the characters themselves in the chapter called "The Syndromes." I want to tell you about the pudgy guy who's just let himself go; the former athlete who just can't stop competing; the skinny gal who's running 50 miles a week, hoping that the fat lady she

1

used to be won't catch up with her; the 48 year-old thrill seeker whose character development stalled somewhere back in the sixties; the vain body builder who never met a mirror he didn't like; and the "life-altering-events" that bring all of them in to see me. I guarantee you know these people. Hell, you may BE these people. After you meet these characters, we'll systematically go through the common orthopedic problems that I treat, region by region. I bet you will see yourself there as well—probably over and over.

So that you can follow the discussion, I'll first teach you to speak like an orthopedist by introducing you to the "lingo" that we doctors use to confuse the enemy. Soon you'll know where the medial side of your knee is and where the distal end of your radius ought to be. You'll be able to hold your own when your doctor says you have "osteoarthritis" or "degenerative disc disease," or worse yet, a "synovial process."

I will give you a tour of the various bones and joints, one by one, because each is so specialized, each reacts in its own way to injury and each has its own story. Within each anatomic region we'll look at how the conditions and injuries that afflict boomers are unique and, at least in part, avoidable. In a sense, this book is an operating manual for the musculoskeletal system. In it I describe all your moving parts and how they work together. I even discuss where to get replacement parts if you need them, but, more importantly, I offer some sensible strategies for their maintenance and repair.

Did you ever wonder why exercise is good for you, but why too much of the wrong kind of exercise is bad? How you are supposed to figure out how much is too much, and under what conditions? Do you have questions about whether exercise is helpful or harmful for arthritis—or whether too much of the wrong type of exercise might even *cause* arthritis? Does it make sense to you that the same exercise or sport you were able to enjoy at twenty-something may be hazardous to your health at fifty-something? If man is the "crown of creation," then why do 80% of us have back pain? I'll answer these questions and many others, based on my experiences with thousands of patients.

I will discuss openly the pros and cons of surgery and how we make decisions recommending or discouraging it. Did you know that despite some miraculous technical advances such as joint replacement and less invasive arthroscopic surgeries, we are still the victims of our own technology? Do you know what operations are bad for you more often than good for you? How do you know when your surgeon is recommending surgery because it's the best treatment and not just because—well, he's a surgeon? How can you avoid having unrealistic expectations of technology?

I am a "general" orthopedic surgeon, which means that I see and treat most orthopedic conditions and all of the age groups from cradle to grave. For the last twenty-eight years, I have treated fractures, arthroscoped knees, done around a hundred joint replacements a year, treated back aches and sore feet, operated on hands and wiggled little baby hips to see if they are hooked up right. Most orthopods in this country are like me: general orthopedists with some specialty training or interest. I may do more hips, knees, hands and shoulders than the others in my group, but I don't swallow my tongue when someone walks in with a bunion or a pinched nerve in the neck. The sub-specialist who does just hands or hips or pediatrics is the exception, not the rule.

I trained at two of the premier orthopedic institutions in the country: the University of Iowa College of Medicine in my hometown of Iowa City, Iowa, and the Mayo Clinic in Rochester, Minnesota where I did my orthopedic residency. I've been in private practice in a small city in Southeast Iowa, the Chairman of Orthopedics at the largest teaching hospital in the Air Force and am now the Residency Program Director at the Ochsner Clinic in New Orleans. I've taken care of too many broken hips to count, operated on casualties fresh off the battlefield, and watched teenagers I operated on grow up and go to medical school. In my current job, I am not only in charge of the training of twelve orthopedic residents, but I'm also the Chairman of Graduate Medical Education for the 250-some doctors we have training in twenty-five residencies and fellowships at our institution. Though I've spent most of my career in academic medicine and in large hospitals, I never forget that I started private practice at age twenty-eight as one of only three orthopedists in a community of 40,000.

So, if you're like most boomers, you're very interested in what makes you tick and you'll keep reading. In this book you, my friend, are the star of the show; but remember that's a double-edged sword. I intend to upset some of your cherished assumptions and to present in their place, more sensible ways of maintaining your musculoskeletal system. If you've ever had a backache, sprained an ankle, or dislocated your shoulder, you can turn to that chapter and get some answers. More importantly, though, I want to teach you why orthopedists think the way we think. In that process I'm going to have to divulge some professional secrets. I promise to keep it entertaining, but somehow that's easier when the subject, the audience and the author are one and the same. This is a book *of* the boomers, *by* a boomer and *for* the boomers.

Chapter 1: The Syndromes

I've watched my fellow baby boomers age with me, some more gracefully than others. Their problems and their complaints fall into the usual anatomic categories (problems of the back, the shoulder, the knee etc.), but also into certain themes, which I like to call "The Syndromes." That's one of those words doctors use to confuse the enemy. "Syndrome" is really just a ten-dollar word for a cluster of symptoms or a recurring theme that keeps showing up in your office. Before taking on each of the common problems that affect the anatomic regions, I'd like to discuss some of those themes that cross the typical anatomic boundaries. These are the syndromes that set us apart as baby boomers, at least as far as they affect the musculoskeletal system.

The Syndrome of Deconditioning

The most common syndrome is the harried, 45-year-old man or woman who is "deconditioned". It is no secret that more of us are out of shape than are fit. No matter how much they drummed gym class into us when we were kids, no matter how many presidents committed their administrations to the health and fitness of America's youth, we are, in the majority, a bunch of slobs. We may waver between guilt and determination, committing every now and then to a program of fitness and healthy living, but in the end entropy wins out and we slouch and snack our way into big blobs of

5

mostly fat and wind held together by anxiety. We call this state "deconditioning."

The musculoskeletal system is either a lousy design or a remarkably flexible, adaptable design, depending on your perspective and mostly depending on your maintenance of it. In that sense, it's like a fine racing bicycle: when everything is all tuned, the cables are tight and you're in shape to ride it, nothing seems more well suited to the task of covering the ground ahead. On the other hand, if the wheels are out of alignment, the sprockets rusty, the handlebars loose and the rider's butt way outsized for the racing seat, it's a rolling comedy with a tragedy around the next corner.

The skeleton and its muscles were originally "designed" with a horizontal spine suspended between four limbs, with two before, and two aft, not to mention a tail and few other handy things. As we evolved from our arboreal ancestors, we rose to walk on those hind limbs, freeing the hands to get into all sorts of mischief (some would include orthopedic surgery here), forever dooming the spine, the shoulders, the knees and their supporting cast of muscles to a lifetime of playing from behind. The model that we now drive is woefully under-designed for the world in which we currently live. It also was not meant to function more than about four or maybe five decades. How many 70-year-old apes do you know? So, it's no wonder that we should start to see the cumulative effect of those design flaws, of that unexpected longevity and of our own poor maintenance—*and* that we should start to creak at about our age.

On the other hand, you have all seen some vintage car that has been cherished by its owner, only driven on sunny days and hand-rubbed to a glossy sheen, cruising by all proud and stately. With only a little maintenance, a little attention to detail and some loving care, the human musculoskeletal system can cruise us into the seventh, eighth and even ninth decade in pretty good shape. You may need a new fuel pump or a tire change along the way, but surely a complete lack of maintenance will have the predictable effect we call deconditioning.

The deconditioned patient comes into the orthopedic clinic looking for some quick fix to what is, in fact, the final failure of some part or system of parts that have gone without maintenance for a lifetime. Surgery is the preferred answer. He wants to hear that I have some procedure that will whisk away the pain and erase five decades of self-abuse. When you're 100 pounds overweight (and where I live some 20% of us are!) the question is not "Why does my knee hurt, Doc?" The question is "Well, how could you expect that knee to hold up under that weight for as long as it did?" Still, boomers want to get it "fixed" and get back to the office, back on the road, or back home. They don't want to hear about weight loss or anti-inflammatory medicines, and certainly not exercise that they have to do for themselves. In fact, many don't want to hear about anything that they have to do for themselves. They would prefer something be *done to* them, much like you'd take a car in and leave it with the mechanic, then come back later and drive it away.

The syndrome of deconditioning affects all the parts of the musculoskeletal system but the symptoms are found primarily in the spine, both the neck and lower back, the shoulders and the knees. I'll speak specifically about each of these later.

The "Fitness-is-Competition" Syndrome

Another syndrome is what I call *"fitness is competition."* Not all members of our generation are slobs and couch potatoes. Many are avid athletes who really bought into all that sports stuff when they were kids. These were often the stars in gym class; the natural athletes who participated in varsity athletics, the letter jacket guys with all the chicks. Sans the chicks, I was one of these characters. We were the ones who were at the head of your little squad leading the calisthenics, the first to be chosen for that pick-up basketball game, and the guys who either went on to play sports in college or maybe played on an intramural team for their company. These are the jocks.

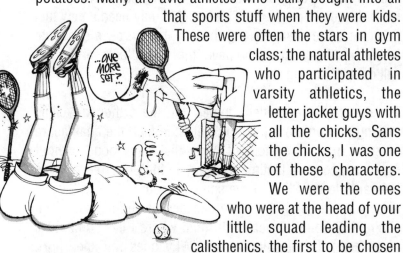

The problem for the jocks is that somewhere in the brain fitness got associated, or rather confused, with competition. For some this association becomes so pernicious that they are only happy when they are whipping somebody's butt. These guys don't jog unless they are training for a road race. They prefer those one-on-one, mano-a-mano sports like racquetball, squash or better yet, handball. "Just give me a ball, a wall and somebody I can beat up on; that's all I ask. That's how I'll stay fit." Some drift into team sports like basketball, volleyball, or softball, but even then, they prefer smaller pick-up games, two-on-two, half-court, in-your-face competition. The idea of swimming or walking on a treadmill with some headphones on just doesn't appeal to these guys. And here I use the term guys in the male gender, because this is almost solely a male syndrome.

As these competitive jocks age, they are prone to injuries, many of them serious, like torn cruciate ligaments in the knee, torn rotator cuffs in the shoulder, ruptured Achilles tendons etc. When age and injury (or sometimes surgery) take away their ability to compete, they know of no other satisfying way to stay fit. They go into whip-your-butt withdrawal and the whole house of cards comes crashing down.

Recent statistics have identified just how serious this syndrome is and how commonly boomers are injuring themselves in sporting pursuits. There is even a new name for this: "Boomeritis." Recently the American Academy of Orthopedic Surgeons has published the following shocking data. Those of us born between 1946 and 1964 will suffer more than one million sports-related injuries this year. The estimated cost of treating these injuries will exceed 18 billion dollars. There were 33% more sports-related injuries in 1998 than in 1991. This led to over 365,000 Boomers carted into the nation's emergency rooms in 1998 alone. The most common sports involved were bicycling, basketball, skiing and exercise and running. This is clearly an emerging problem, if not yet an epidemic.

The "Fear-of-becoming-the-fat-lady" Syndrome

Then there's the interesting female gender-specific syndrome, *"I'm thin now, but there's a fat lady running right behind me."* This syndrome kind of ties together the first two. Here you have before you what appears to be a fit women who has just pushed her body to the point of breakdown, and sometimes literally to the point of what we call "fatigue (or stress) fracture." She may be running 30 miles a week, jogging hours every day on the treadmill or maybe bounding around in two different step-aerobics classes, one before work and one after. She might have leg pain that turns out to be a bone Jazzersized to the point of breaking, or maybe kneecaps that can no longer climb umpteen thousand flights on the StairMaster after work everyday. But on closer examination you will find that she used to be fat.

FASTER... FASTER... FASTER...

YOOO-HOOO!

Sometimes she was really fat. And what's going on here is that although the woman before you is as thin as a jeans ad, she's got this fat lady jiggling along behind her. And if she ever stops . . . well, that fat lady's going to catch her.

These women respond with the same incredulous look as the jocks when I suggest that the treatment for what ails them is rest from their routine, substitution of some less sexy fitness program, rehab of the abused part and then gradual resumption of their activities—but never to the level of self-abuse that they previously treasured.

The Risk Takers

Next there are the *"risk takers."* These are the nostalgics who remember the fun of plunging headlong down the hill on a Schwinn Flyer, tobogganing down the snowy run in the dark, or hitchhiking across Europe with a 50-pound backpack. They remember what it was like to be 10 and maybe 20 but have not yet come to grips with being 45 or 50. I see these people every winter as they limp back to New Orleans from the ski slopes, or are air-evacuated up from some Caribbean Island where they damn near drowned

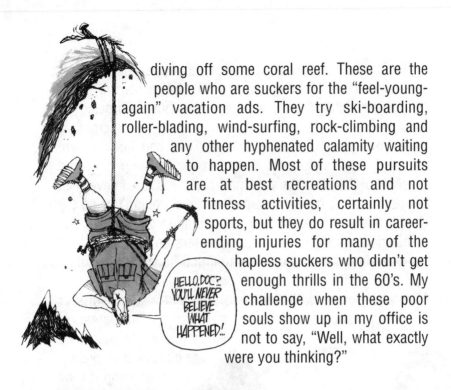

diving off some coral reef. These are the people who are suckers for the "feel-young-again" vacation ads. They try ski-boarding, roller-blading, wind-surfing, rock-climbing and any other hyphenated calamity waiting to happen. Most of these pursuits are at best recreations and not fitness activities, certainly not sports, but they do result in career-ending injuries for many of the hapless suckers who didn't get enough thrills in the 60's. My challenge when these poor souls show up in my office is not to say, "Well, what exactly were you thinking?"

The Narcissus Syndrome

This is my term for the self-absorbed fascination we have with our own bodies. Here boomers succumb to the constant barrage of advertising pressure to look like something out of a Greek sculpture garden. This syndrome affects both sexes. I'm no Greek scholar, but I have called this the "Narcissus Syndrome" after the character in mythology that fell in love with his own reflection in the pool. We somehow get suckered into thinking that we're all supposed to have 10% body fat, big well-defined muscles, the waistline of a snake, the hair of Ronald Reagan and the smile of a Pepsodent ad. Spectacles, potbellies, and yellow teeth simply don't fit into this picture. Boomers will go to great lengths to rework themselves into this image, as if we're all supposed to be Michelangelo's David or a *Baywatch* babe.

Patients who fit this syndrome work out not for the exercise or the fitness, but almost purely for the physical appearance. The term "body building" says it all. Notice it's not called "body remodeling," as if we were somehow improving on what we've already got, but rather starting from scratch. I have taken care of body-builders who had such severe carpal tunnel syndrome from weight-training that the muscles of their thumbs were partially paralyzed. I have seen the nerve to the hand so damaged that it couldn't bring the thumb across the palm. Yet, they wouldn't stop lifting. The discussion leading up to surgery centers on how soon after the operation they could return to lifting how much weight.

Men and women with this syndrome will take all sorts of supplements and hormones. The latest is testosterone for men who are building their bodies. There's going to be a testosterone gel, now available in France, out on the U.S. market soon. This is testosterone that penetrates the skin without all the needles or pills. You watch; guys will be smearing this stuff all over like sunscreen. Patients will rarely give their doctor a history of taking these chemicals. They may be squeamish because what they have been ingesting is either frankly illegal or, at best, a spurious application of a drug with a legitimate use, like growth hormone. Sometimes they just think because these are "nutritional supplements" that they are somehow "natural." The androstenedione used by baseball slugger Mark McGuire is an example in this category. Natural is fine as long as you're willing to accept a few side effects like generalized acne, an enlarged prostate, tiny testicles and a drop in HDL—the good kind of cholesterol.

The orthopedic complications of all this vanity usually affect the muscles and the tendons. Narcissus gets a ruptured biceps tendon or some other muscle strain, like rotator cuff tendonitis in the shoulder. When these patients come in to see me, they want to know what they can do to get over this latest setback in their body building regimen so that they can get back to training. Here I have to admit that I just don't have that "Sports Medicine" mentality. It seems to me that if you've damaged your shoulder lifting too much unnecessary weight—say bench-pressing over 300 pounds—you should be willing to back off on that amount of weight for a while. You may even need to stop lifting completely for a time, and substitute some less stressful regimen that involves lighter weights and more repetitions instead. But this recommendation is usually met with skepticism because these guys are not going for endurance. They are sculptors, pure and simple, and they will only see results with large weights lifted until failure. Unfortunately, it is exactly that failure that brings them to see me. This syndrome is not limited to patients, by the way. I've had orthopedic residency candidates (doctors who want to train to become orthopedists) and at least one guy who interviewed for a job with us, send pictures of themselves lifting weights or otherwise flexing for the cameras. I'm still waiting for someone to send me an MRI of his bulging brain, which would seem a more appropriate way to impress me.

The Life-Altering Event

Finally, there's the syndrome of the "Life-Altering Event," or LAE for short. This can arise from any of the other syndromes but in all cases it involves somehow losing balance. The risk taker might take that Black Diamond run on the last afternoon of the last day of his lift ticket, hit that tree and WHAM! An LAE. The deconditioned office worker might decide now's the time to get back into shape, run a few too many blocks and drop over with that coronary. The 50-year-old jock might go one-on-one with that 20-year-old kid in the gym and OOPS! There goes his anterior cruciate ligament for good. The once-was-a-fat-lady might run and run some more on that treadmill, ignoring that groin pain that is actually heralding a stress fracture of her hip until CRACK! Another one bites the dust.

These are all examples of a life-altering event. Nobody really wants to take the time out to have surgery, go through the rehabilitation, the pain and grief, the lost time at work, all for something that was essentially preventable. No one is ever quite the same after tearing his ACL or fracturing her hip or having the Big One. We are a generation of over-doers. We work too hard, play way too hard, drink too heavily, did too many drugs in the past and seem collectively incapable of moderation. We should be careful not to let our dramatically over-sized sense of self get us in trouble. We should be a little more careful, take fewer physical risks and work more toward balance in our physical fitness and recreational pursuits. I know this sounds a lot more like philosophy than orthopedics but, believe me, most people would rather have an appointment with the philosopher than with the orthopedic surgeon.

My advice is that anytime you can feel the wind in your hair, you're probably perilously close to an LAE. Not that you shouldn't go ride your bike, but wear a helmet, OK?

Though not all the orthopedic patients our age come to me with one or more of these syndromes, they are collectively so common that any discussion of the usual anatomic problems would be incomplete without this background. There is almost always more than meets the eye to these injuries, or, in this case, more than meets the shoulder or the knee or the back. And these syndromes represent part of the context in which many other afflictions arise . . . a context unique to baby boomers.

Chapter 2: The Lingo— Anatomic Terminology

I've always loved jargon. Every profession has its jargon, those "inside" phrases that put the user in the know and keep everybody else on the outside. Jargon is by nature segregationist; it separates those with the keys to the kingdom from those without. No profession uses this exclusionary language more than medicine. We use it like the French use their language: to talk openly in front of outsiders without them having the slightest idea what we're saying. In the old days doctors used Latin to communicate secretly with each other and to a lesser extent to talk across other language barriers. Some of those old Latin usages persist. For instance, in modern prescription writing, "P.O." is the abbreviation for something taken orally, taken from the Latin "per os" that is, by mouth. The left eye is "O.S." to the ophthalmologist, taken from the Latin "oculus sinister," and so on. We could write "by mouth", I suppose, but where's the fun in that?

Then we have dialects within the profession where, much like the Irish talking to the Australians, they can understand each other, but only with some difficulty. There is a certain basic vocabulary that all doctors understand and share. But for an orthopedist to listen to a cardiologist talking about heart rhythm problems is much like a guy from Liverpool asking directions of someone from the ninth ward in New Orleans. There's some common ground there, but just as likely even more confusion.

This gets more complicated when the doctor gropes for a common language with the patient to whom he's trying to explain the finer points of say, chondromalacia patella. The conversation often goes something like this.

> *Doc*: "Well Jennifer, what you've got here is a chondral defect on the articular surface of your patella. This has probably arisen partly from your excessive femoral anteversion and exaggerated valgus knee angle."

> *Jennifer*: "Oh? And exactly what does all that mean?"

> *Doc*: "Well, it means that the smooth joint surface on the underside of your kneecap is slightly worn out from too much pressure. That goes back to the way you're built; a little too much knock-knee."

> *Jennifer*: "Oh, is there anything you can do about that?"

> *Doc*: "Actually, no. But it sure is fun to talk about it."

I watch this verbal disconnect going on all the time. I'll walk in the room and hear my resident going over the consent for total hip replacement, casually expounding on the "acetabular component" when the patient *might* understand it if he'd said "hip socket." As physicians, we eventually learn to tailor our conversation to the patient's lingua franca and not our own jargon. This takes some practice but after a while one learns that it is in everyone's best interest if we establish some common language. We may think we're all speaking English, but we have to set out some mutual definitions or you won't understand what I'm trying to get across.

When it comes to anatomic terminology in this book, I'm going to try to confine my jargon to a few cardinal directions, and the names for a few anatomic regions (which may not be exactly in keeping with what your mother taught you in the tub). Wherever necessary, I'll give you simple drawings. I like to draw and I find it's one of the quickest ways to get a point across in the clinic. A little artistic talent (and in my case *very little* artistic talent) goes a long way toward helping a patient visualize what I'm talking about.

The Cardinal Directions

Growing up in the Midwest, everything is north, south, east or west. Those are the cardinal directions on the two-dimensional grid that is the Great Plains. If you have any question, just get out of map of Iowa and you'll see roads that go straight this way and straight that way. New Orleans, on the other hand, is quite different. Here the Mississippi River winds along in a snake-like west to east meander that makes those midwestern cardinal directions meaningless. Here the cardinal directions are uptown, downtown, riverside and lakeside. A street corner that in Iowa City would be called the northwest corner of Linn and Brown Streets, here becomes the uptown-lakeside corner of St. Charles and Carrolton.

The human body is three-dimensional, so we need coordinates that describe locations in those three directions. We call up "superior" and down "inferior." Here's how it works. Anything toward the head is said to be superior to anything toward the feet. Anything toward the feet is said to be inferior to anything toward the head. So the belly button is in the middle, but superior to the knees and inferior to the shoulders. The chin is superior to the neck, yet inferior to the eyes and so on. Just like on a map, these are relative terms. The west coast of the United States is still east of Hawaii.

The front of the body is called "anterior" and the back parts are called "posterior." The belly button is anterior to the spine and shoulder blade is posterior to the breast. This is pretty easy to remember in that almost everyone has heard the butt referred to as one's "posterior."

The last cardinal axis is going from side to side; things toward the midline of the body are said to be "medial" and things away from the middle are said to be "lateral." Thus, the knee has a medial side (that part that's closest to the other knee) and a lateral side (that part that's toward the outside, or farthest from the other knee).

Just like we combine the cardinal map directions into northeast and southwest, we combine these anatomic directions into "superomedial" and "posterolateral," and so forth. I'll try to avoid these more sophisticated descents into jargon, but if I slip up, cut me some slack. I still tell my friends in New Orleans that I live northwest of the river, even though they have not the slightest idea what I'm talking about.

There are a couple other terms that are useful, though they are not exactly anatomic cardinal directions. We sometimes speak of "peripheral" and "central." These terms mean exactly what they sound like, peripheral circulation being that out toward the ends of the limbs and central circulation being that near the center of the body. Then there are the surgeon's terms "superficial" and "deep." Again these terms are pretty much self-explanatory, with anything toward the surface of the body being superficial to anything below it, which is said to be deep. The skin is superficial to the muscle underneath it, but the bone may be deep to the muscle.

When moving along a limb we often use another pair of relative terms: "proximal" and "distal." Proximal means "near" and distal means "far." Now, exactly why we don't just say the "far end of the limb" instead of the "distal end of the limb" is just another example of playing hard to get, but you will hear me lapse into this frequently. We talk about the "distal interphalangeal joint," for instance, when we designate the last knuckle on any finger.

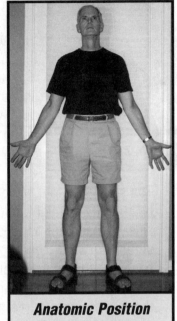

Finally, since the limbs can twist, we establish the convention that all these anatomic terms are taken from the body standing in what we call (get this) "the anatomic position."

In the anatomic position the human body is seen standing, facing the

Anatomic Position

observer with arms at the sides and the hands facing palms forward. This way lateral is officially on the thumb side and medial is officially on the small finger side. Again, I won't try to confuse you, and wherever I can use a simple illustration to make my point I will, but knowing the terms superior, inferior, medial, lateral, anterior and posterior will make it easier for you to follow along.

Regions by Name

What you probably call the arm, I call the "upper extremity." The arm is actually only that part of the upper extremity that goes from the shoulder to the elbow. Below that (or if you want to use the new jargon that you've just learned you

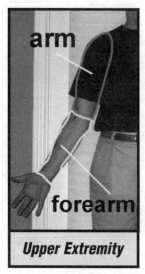

Upper Extremity

could say, "inferior" to that) is the forearm. The upper extremity consists of the *arm* above the elbow and the *forearm* below it.

Similarly, the lower extremity consists of the thigh (above the knee and below the hip) and the leg (below the knee and above the ankle). Inconsistent? You bet, but if you say "leg" to an orthopedist, he's going to think you're talking about only the lower half of the lower extremity.

The spine has four regions. Viewed from head-on it is straight, but viewed from the side, it has four curves. The first one curves forward, the second one curves back, the third curves forward again, and the fourth curves back again. The neck is the first forward curve and is called the "cervical spine." The second part of the spine is that part to which the ribs are attached and that houses the lungs, the heart and the great vessels. It's called the "thoracic spine." That bothersome third part, which we think of as the lower back, curves slightly forward again and is without ribs. We call it the "lumbar spine." Finally, the last segment of the spine curves backward again and in humans is fused into one bony triangular mass that is the cornerstone of the pelvis. This is called the "sacrum."

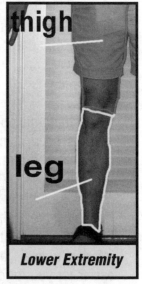

Lower Extremity

Tissue Terminology

As orthopedists, we tend to talk as if everyone else has read the same operating manual and committed all the terms to memory. This is especially true when we start throwing around the names of all the various tissues we deal with: muscle, tendon, ligament, cartilage etc. Though I can expect almost everyone to know what I mean when I say "bone," beyond that, the assumption that we share any working understanding of these tissue definitions breaks down. You may know that muscle is the stuff you are eating when you ingest "meat," but, then again, you may not really want to think about that. When I tell you that you have "torn a muscle," you probably don't equate this with ruining lunch.

So let's identify the basic tissue types that make up the musculoskeletal system.

Bone

This one should be easy. Anybody who's ever eaten chicken has worked with examples of long bones, flat bones and all the other tissues we'll be talking about. Bone is a remarkable tissue. For a detailed description of its qualities, please refer to *Chapter 12: Fractures of the Long Bones.* Bone is both the structural element that gives the human

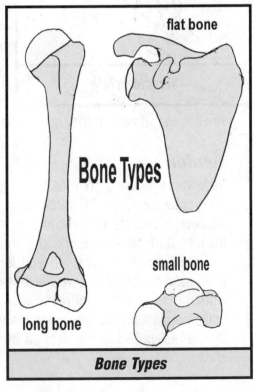

Bone Types

Bone Types

body form and support, and the tissue that creates the protective housing for its most precious parts: the brain and the vital organs. Everyone knows a bone when they see one.

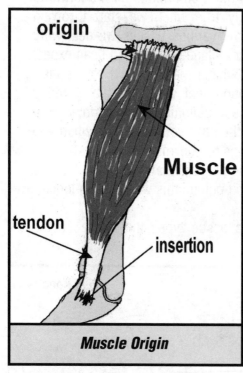

origin

Muscle

tendon

insertion

Muscle Origin

Muscle

Muscle is the next easiest tissue to recognize because, again, we've seen it and we frequently eat it. What I call "skeletal muscle," you call barbecue. Muscles are the motors that move the skeleton by contracting and acting across a moveable joint. Muscles are dynamic; use them and they get better at what they do. They can get stronger and bigger, if they need to, and they will get smaller and wimpier if they are not used.

Tendon

Now we're starting to move away from the familiar. Not everyone knows that a tendon is that bit of fibrous tissue that anchors a muscle to whatever it moves or pulls on. The muscle and tendon work together as what we call a "musculo-tendinous unit." If you look at your wrist on the palm side of your hand, you will see a bunch of tendons at work. The muscle contracts, the tendon at its end is pulled proximally as the muscle shortens, and the joint it crosses is moved in the desired direction. That's how they work together as a unit. Tendons themselves do not change in length during this process. They are straps of a fixed length, pulled in a given direction by a specific muscle with a specific job to do—flex the wrist, extend the knee or hold up the head.

Origin and Insertion

Muscles have a beginning and an end, and we have a name for each. The place where a muscle starts is called its "origin" and the place where its tendon attaches is called its "insertion." A few muscles have tendons at both the origin and the insertion, but most have a broader origin and a smaller tendinous insertion. For example, the muscle that extends your wrist has its origin off the humerus, above the elbow and inserts as a tendon onto one of the bones on the back of the hand.

Ligament

Ligaments are often confused with tendons, partly because they are made of exactly the same kind of fibrous tissue. But ligaments are the straps that hold the joints together. Ligaments go from one point on a bone, cross a joint and then attach to another point on another bone.

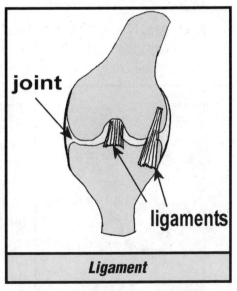

Ligament

Ligaments are static. They keep a joint from going too far in an undesirable direction. Whereas a tendon is moving when its muscle is acting, a ligament stays put, holding its joint together.

Strains and Sprains

One reason that ligaments and tendons are often confused is that the names we give an injury to either sound so much alike. An injury to a musculo-tendinous unit is a "strain" and an injury to a ligament is called a "sprain." Quite a few medical professionals don't get this right and these terms get murdered all the time, so let's get this straight. You can *strain* your biceps muscle, or *strain* your Achilles tendon, but you can't *sprain* either. You can *sprain* your anterior cruciate ligament or *sprain* your lateral ankle ligaments, but you cannot *strain* them.

Still with me? OK . . .

Joint

Anywhere two bones get together, they are "joined" at an articulation that we call a joint. These joints may not move at all, they may move a little or they may move a lot, but they all share certain characteristics. They involve at least two bones, they are restrained by ligaments, and they have some sort of specialized tissue on the end of the bones that interact at the joint.

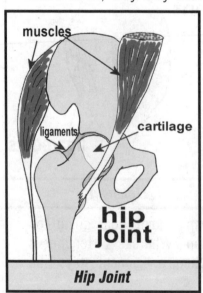

Hip Joint

The most typical joints are those that move a lot. I'll use the hip as an example. The hip is a simple ball and socket arrangement with a round ball at the upper end of the femur, fitting closely into a reciprocal round cup in the pelvis. This joint is restrained by strong ligaments that pass from the neck of the femur to the edge of the socket. The hip joint is moved by strong muscles that pass over it in all directions.

Inside the joint, the bone ends are covered with another remarkable tissue we call "cartilage." This "articular" or joint cartilage is a very specialized tissue that absorbs shocks, provides an incredibly smooth bearing surface and even participates in its own lubrication. It is so specialized that, like brain tissue, it has almost completely given up its ability to heal. This is a truism: the more sophisticated or specialized the tissue, the harder it is for it to heal or regenerate. The same can be said for doctors, by the way. The more specialized we get, the harder it is to do what might be considered basic functions. I've seen orthopedists use a stethoscope as a tendon hammer, for instance.

You've seen this articular cartilage too, though you may not have noticed it. If you take that chicken wing and break it open at the joint, the yellow-gray smooth stuff on the ends of the bones is articular cartilage.

Now I'm going to complicate things a little, because it turns out there is more than one type of cartilage. Though "articular cartilage" is what we usually mean when we say "cartilage," the knee has another kind of cartilage we call

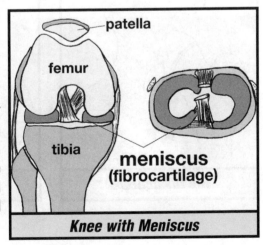

patella
femur
tibia
meniscus
(fibrocartilage)

Knee with Meniscus

"fibro-cartilage." This makes up the famous meniscus.

When we speak of someone having "torn a cartilage" in the knee, we're referring to a tear in this little washer of gristle. Fibro-cartilage is nothing like articular cartilage and I wish we called it something else, but beware! The knee has both articular cartilage and the fibro-cartilage menisci, so it can become confusing. To make it even worse, degeneration of both is involved in the process we call arthritis.

Joint injuries may involve sprains that injure the ligaments or more severe injuries we call "dislocations" and "subluxations." A complete loss of joint congruity is called a dislocation. Again using the hip as an example, when the ball is completely out of the socket, it is called a hip dislocation. When the ball is only partly out of the socket, it is called a subluxation. These are matters of degree, with the dislocation being the more serious injury.

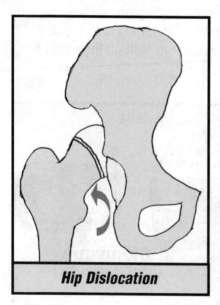

Hip Dislocation

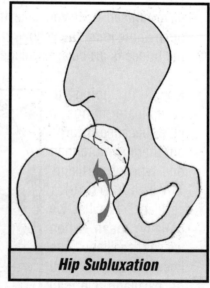

Hip Subluxation

Fracture Terminology

Because I will be talking about fractures that occur in all the anatomic regions, it will be helpful to define some of the common terms used in talking about fractures and their treatment.

First, a fracture is any loss of the structural or functional integrity of the bone. This definition includes the obvious, catastrophic failures, but also includes stress fractures and other conditions that might not show complete disruption of the bone on the x-ray. As long as the bone is unable to do its main job, then it is considered fractured. A stress fracture of the metatarsal bone in the foot, for instance, may not even show up on an x-ray, and yet the patient can't bear weight.

When a fractured bone is out of place, we call the act of setting it, "reducing" the fracture. Thus, fracture reduction means getting the fractured ends of the bone back into an acceptable alignment. This may be done without opening up the fracture, in which case it is called a "closed reduction." If I have to open the fracture surgically to fix it, it is called an "open reduction." If I leave a bunch of hardware (pins, plates or screws) behind, this is called "open reduction and internal fixation." This is affectionately abbreviated, ORIF.

ORIF

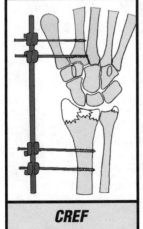

CREF

Some fractures can be reduced closed but must be held in place with pins that we put in without opening the fracture and that are held apart with an external frame we call an "external fixiter." This makes for an operation we call "closed reduction and external fixation" or CREF.

Not all fractures heal properly or promptly, and we have a lingo to describe that too. We call the process of fracture healing "union," so that a fracture that doesn't heal is called a "non-union." A fracture that is slow to heal is called a "delayed union." A fracture that heals in an unacceptable position is called a "mal-union."

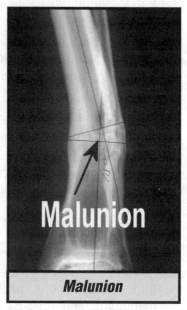

Malunion

Please don't get discouraged. I know this chapter sounds like the first day of some foreign language class. As we get deeper into the discussion of various problems in the boomer musculoskeletal system, I promise to define new terms as I introduce them, so that we can all keep on the same page and keep speaking the same language. I hope you find this more fun that confusing, but if you lose your directions, you can refer back to this chapter and it should help you to catch up.

Chapter 3: Arthritis

The Most Common Type of Arthritis: Osteoarthritis (OA)

If you walk down the aisle at Barnes and Noble looking for a book on arthritis and its treatment, you might come away thinking it's either a deficiency of flax seed, or caused by too little yoga. And you might think it can be treated with everything from cobalt salts to miracle extracts. A patient comes into my office at least once a month and sheepishly unfolds a tattered article clipped from some magazine or newspaper, expounding the latest cure for arthritis. "Doc, what do you think of this?" What I want to say is, "Well, do you believe in Tinkerbell?" But I usually explain that this is yet another magical elixir in the long tradition of snake oil. As Abe said, "You can fool all of the people some of the time and some of the people all of the time…" I don't want you to be fooled at all. In this chapter I'm going to try to straighten out what arthritis is, what it isn't, and what can and can't be done about it.

I'm going to make four key points. First, osteoarthritis is not a single disease, but the final common pathway of joint failure from any of a number of causes. Second, osteoarthritis is not just a joint cartilage problem. Third, there is not now and will not be in the near future, a cure for osteoarthritis. Finally, in order not to get snookered, you need to know what actually works in the treatment of arthritis—and what hasn't been proven to work.

Mythology: The Cause and the Cure

If we ever find a "cure" for arthritis, it's going to put a lot of us out of business. Joint failure is such a universal human experience that it is often attributed to simple aging, but that view is incomplete. It is true that osteoarthritis becomes more common as we age, but it is not inevitable or even symmetrical. Why do some people have just one hip or one knee go bad? Presumably the other hip is the same age and has been along for the same ride. In our culture we have a way of looking for some one thing to blame. We long to believe that our arthritis has a cause—that football injury 20 years ago. I think for boomers it's just more acceptable to be wounded than to be wearing out. Recently I had a 350-pound patient in my office with a completely worn out knee, and he wanted to blame his arthritis on some fall he took 30 years before. He was dead certain that slip and fall had more to do with his pain and suffering than the cumulative damage of being two times his ideal body weight for his entire adult life.

The truth is, arthritis is not one disease at all. Though there are many variations, arthritis comes in two basic types. The great divide in arthritis falls between the more common degenerative condition we call "osteoarthritis" and the group of inflammatory arthritides typified by rheumatoid arthritis. We will consider each separately. Although there is some overlap, the underlying mechanisms of these two types of arthritis are quite distinct. I'll start with the more common diagnosis: osteoarthritis.

Don't Tell Me It's Just Arthritis!

I've probably spent more time in my career explaining what osteoarthritis is, and what it isn't, than in any other conversation I have with my patients. Americans seem to think that arthritis is some sort of minor problem, a little nuisance that, though irritating, should go away with Tylenol (acetaminophen) or Advil (ibuprofen). In fact, osteoarthritis is a chronic, progressive, often crippling condition. It is the main reason orthopedic surgeons do over half a million total hip and knee replacements in this country every year. Yet patients commonly are shocked and even disappointed to find out that what is wrong with them is "just arthritis."

"What do you mean it's *just arthritis*, doctor? How could that be? I'm in such pain! Don't try to tell me that it is *just arthritis!*"

Well, *just arthritis* is enough to force you to use a cane, or even crutches, keep you from sleeping, or steal your ability to walk from point A to point B. When it affects your hands it may make the simplest activity either miserable or impossible. I see 50-year-old women who can't open a pill bottle and guys my age (52) who can't button a shirt button. When it affects the shoulder it may keep you from lifting your hand over your head, make getting into a t-shirt impossible, or it may force you to sleep sitting up. The predilection of osteoarthritis for the spine, particularly the low back, is one of the universal miseries of mankind and the most common reason for Americans to miss work or become permanently disabled. But still we don't want to hear that it's *just arthritis*.

Joints Most Commonly Affected By OA
• Spine • Hips • Knees • Hands

Osteoarthritis has several aliases, and I suppose each is an attempt to give this condition a more palatable or more descriptive name. We sometimes call osteoarthritis, "degenerative arthritis," implying that there is some underlying wear and tear process that sneaks up on the joint, causing it to fail. Some patients seem to like the term "degenerative." Patients tell me all the time that they've been told they have a "degenerative condition," or that they have "cartilage degeneration," as if somehow that way of putting it is more glamorous than "just arthritis." But it's all the same thing.

Point #1: Osteoarthritis Is Not a Single Disease, But Joint Failure from Any Cause.

It is more useful to understand end-stage osteoarthritis as organ failure in which the organ that fails is the joint. When your kidneys fail, you might go on dialysis and eventually, if you're lucky, get a kidney transplant. When your heart fails, same thing, only there's no equivalent of dialysis for a bum ticker. It's either straight to a transplant or straight to the morgue. When your knee fails, it's a slower process, which we call osteoarthritis. Don't be frightened by that statement: not all joint damage will end in joint failure, and we're going to talk about what you can do to prevent or at least slow this process. But in the end, it is that joint failure that can lead to total knee replacement—the orthopedic equivalent of an organ transplant. Osteoarthritis can result from damage, injury or even inherited weakness in any of the structural components that have to work together for the knee to be healthy. Osteoarthritis is the final common pathway for many conditions, but in the end they result in failure of that organ we call the joint.

The joint is a complex organ made up of many interacting parts. Let's look at a common joint and use it to illustrate how many different insults can lead to osteoarthritis.

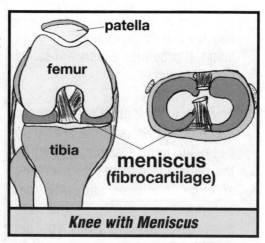

Knee with Meniscus

The knee is that joint in which the end of the thigh bone (femur) and the leg bone (tibia) come together. Each of the bones involved in this joint is covered with a very specialized tissue called articular cartilage. This articular or "joint" cartilage absorbs shocks, provides an incredibly smooth bearing surface, and even participates in its own lubrication. It is so specialized that, like brain tissue, it has almost completely given up its ability to heal. But the knee is even more sophisticated than other joints in that it has another kind of cartilage structure we call the meniscus. The menisci (there are two in each knee) are made up of fibrocartilage, which is much like the gristle of the chicken breast bone or the cartilage framework of your ear or nose. These little washers act as shock absorbers, working in concert with the articular cartilage to spread over a broader surface the impact of walking. This joint is held together by ligaments, firm straps of collagen tissue that run from bone to bone, restraining the motions of the knee as it goes about its business—which is locomotion.

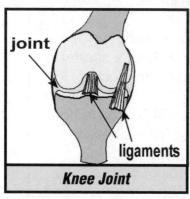

Knee Joint

There are strong muscles that cross the joint, providing the engine for the many remarkable movements and all those steps we take for granted day in and day out. Finally, this whole joint-organ is enclosed in a balloon

35

bag we call the synovium[1], or joint lining. It produces a lubricant called synovial fluid.

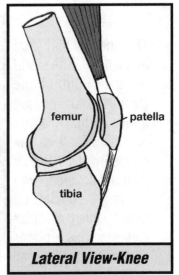

Any significant injury to any of these major components of the knee joint can result in osteoarthritis. Fracture the bone and damage its overlying articular cartilage and you get arthritis. Tear a meniscus and have it removed and eventually you get arthritis. Tear the anterior cruciate ligament, rendering the knee unstable, and the eventual outcome is, guess what? You got it—arthritis. Get an infection in the joint that digests that articular cartilage, or overwhelm the joint with the irritating crystals that form in gout and you have the same thing. So the name of the game is *prevention* of these damaging insults through healthy joint maintenance, avoidance of unnecessary threats to the joints by not participating in risky sports, and early treatment of significant joint injuries to delay the onset of arthritis.

How to Avoid Damage to the Joints That May Lead to OA

- Avoid direct injury to the joint by accident or obesity
- Play it safe when cycling or skiing
- Never go up on a ladder without a spotter
- Avoid competing in sports with much younger athletes
- Don't try to prove you're still 20–you're not!
- Be suspicious of hyphenated recreations (roller-blading, jet-skiing, hang-gliding, para-sailing, bungee-jumping)

1 "Synovium" comes from the Latin words meaning "like the egg white" –syn+ovum. Joint fluid looks and feels like the egg white before it's cooked.

Point #2: OA Is Not Just a
Problem of Articular Cartilage.

This is a critical concept, because patients and physicians alike speak of osteoarthritis as if it is some primary disease process like measles or psoriasis. The implication is that if we could only figure out what caused it, we could cure it. This is as naïve as considering cancer one disease process when, in fact, cancer is no more monolithic than the myriad of different cell types that can go awry. The cancer caused by the cells lining the bladder is nothing like the cancer caused by blood cells or brain cells gone haywire. And just as we won't find some universal cure for all the cancers, we won't find some silver bullet cure for all the things that can lead to osteoarthritis. Grasping this idea helps you understand where we are currently with treatment for osteoarthritis and, hopefully, helps you avoid getting taken by every shyster with the latest potion or—God forbid—operation for arthritis.

I think this misguided notion that OA is somehow just a derangement of the joint cartilage has led a lot of research scientists and clinicians off on a scientific snipe hunt, looking for ways to grow new cartilage, promote its repair, and thereby "cure" osteoarthritis. But if we ignore that torn ligament, that asymmetrically loaded knee joint, the repetitive insults of obesity, the fractured bone below the joint or any of the myriad other causes of joint failure, cartilage repair will never succeed. Even if you could get cartilage cells to shake off their biologically sluggish metabolic habits and get with the program, you would still have to deal with all the other insults that can lead to joint failure. You'd have to prevent everything preventable, reverse everything reversible and manipulate an individual's genetic heritage in order to grab the golden snitch of curing arthritis.

Point #3: There Is Not Now and Will Not Be in the Near Future, a Cure for Osteoarthritis.

So, it boils down to sorting out the science from the snake oil.

I use the knee as an illustration here, but osteoarthritis can affect any joint in the body. It most commonly affects the large weight-bearing joints (the hip and knee), the spine, the hands and the feet. It may be less common in the shoulder and the elbow joint proper, but any injury, especially fractures or dislocations that involve those joints, or any joint infection or systemic condition that damages any joint, can lead to osteoarthritis. A majority of patients over age 65 have OA somewhere, and by age 75, that percentage is over 85%. Women are more likely to be afflicted with OA than men. The silver lining here is that somewhat less than 50% of people who have OA on x-ray experience symptoms.

What is the Natural Progression of Osteoarthritis (OA)?

- Expect arthritis symptoms to have ups and downs, good days and bad.
- Arthritis never completely goes away.
- Arthritis gradually gets worse in most cases, but usually slowly over years.
- Most arthritis can be treated without surgery.

The economic impact of OA is staggering and is estimated to be roughly 30 times that of the other kind of arthritis, rheumatoid arthritis. The wonderful medical textbook published by the Arthritis Foundation, the *Primer of*

Rheumatic Diseases, tenth edition, cites 68 million lost workdays per year for OA versus 2 million for RA.

Osteoarthritis runs in families but, given the demographics, I think one might just as well say that it runs in the Family of Man. You are likely to have your mother's hands and maybe your father's knees. When the 300-pound patient sits in my office carefully cataloguing the minor slips and twists that she thinks must surely have led to her arthritic knee, I usually point out that she might just as well blame her grandmother. You can't change your genetics and you can't stop the clock from ticking, but you can choose a lifestyle that promotes joint health rather than risks damage.

What Should Make You Suspicious You May Have Early OA?

- The Big Three symptoms: pain, swelling, stiffness in a joint
- Previous history of injury to the joint
- Family history of arthritis in the joint ("Mom had knees like these!")
- Asymmetrical joint involvement: right knee, not left knee
- Gradual, insidious onset of symptoms with ups and downs

Symptoms of Osteoarthritis (OA): The "Big Three"

- Pain
- Swelling
- Stiffness of any joint

The symptoms of osteoarthritis are pain, swelling and stiffness. All three symptoms come from the wearing out of the joint. The pain comes from the exposure of bone (which has nerve endings) to abnormal stresses, which in turn comes from the loss of the protective joint cartilage (which has no nerve endings and therefore no feeling). The swelling comes from the joint's reaction to this process, much as if it were trying to make up for the bad bearing by adding lubrication. As the joint wears out, the smooth articular cartilage surface gradually wears down and becomes rough. The body's ability to repair this cartilage is quite limited, and as it wears out the body responds by making more bone at the edge of the joints. These "spurs" at the joint periphery, which we call "osteophytes," are a typical sign of osteoarthritis. Osteophytes are common at the last finger joint. You've all seen women with these little bumpy, sometimes crooked fingers.

Point #4: You Need to Know What Actually Works in the Treatment of Arthritis— and What Hasn't Been Proven to Work.

A lot can be done to make patients with OA feel better. We can prescribe analgesics such as Tylenol (acetaminophen) and the non-steroidal anti-inflammatory drugs (NSAIDs). These drugs are the frontline treatment for palliating the symptoms of pain, swelling and stiffness. We can brace sore joints, splint them, inject them with cortisone and I can point out all the findings on the x-rays 'til the cows come home, but none of these modalities actually influences the natural history of OA. I try to be careful in explaining to patients that we're treating the symptoms and not the condition. None of the arthritis medicines we give does anything to restore the joint. I'll talk about the latest research into "chondro-protective" drugs later, but for now, we have nothing that is really proven to restore cartilage. The only true treatment is *prevention* of joint injury, encouraging joint repair (as we might do by fixing a fracture in the joint) and, in a few cases, surgery to rearrange the evil forces crossing a joint gone crooked. This is precisely what patients find so frustrating. They seem to know that if it is *just arthritis*, we don't have much of anything to offer other than symptom modulation. The good news is that if the joint wears out completely, the operations we have to fix them are among the most effective surgeries out there.

Self-treatment of Osteoarthritis

- Keep your weight down.
- Daily non-impact, aerobic exercise
- Over the counter anti-inflammatories (ibuprofen, naproxen, aspirin)
- Avoid the activities that aggravate symptoms.
- Chondro-protective drugs (chondroitin, glucosamine)

I tell my patients that we really don't have much that we can do surgically in the middle stages of OA. I'm talking as a surgeon here, because patients come in thinking that OA can somehow be controlled so that they experience minimal pain and disability, until the day they wake up and need a knee replacement. Unfortunately, it just doesn't work that way. We recommend sensible, proven effective treatments like weight reduction, isometric strengthening exercises, and non-narcotic analgesics (acetaminophen, ibuprofen and similar drugs). Patients walk out mumbling something like, "If we can put a man on the moon, then why can't we. . .?"

Let's not succumb to that frustration. There really is quite a bit that can be done for the arthritic patient to make him or her feel better, even if those treatments aren't "curing" the disease or making osteoarthritis go away. Let's look at how we can learn to at least live with arthritis. There are several things that you can do for yourself that have a positive influence on the way your arthritis feels and acts. I'll divide these into prevention, nutritional factors and supportive exercise.

"An Ounce of Prevention"

As I said in the *Chapter 1: The Syndromes*, there is currently an epidemic of "sports" related injuries among baby boomers that is being called "Boomeritis". The alarming increase in Emergency Room visits by boomers, who have injured their joints with activities better left to their kids, is preventable. Do you really need to ski that Black Diamond slope or stretch a double by Pete Rose-ing it into third base headfirst? One weekend I was on call I treated a boomer who broke his wrist in just such a move and an accountant who broke his leg playing touch football. I can patch these guys up, but they will lose a great deal of time from work and they may have damaged joints that are now much more likely to develop OA over time than before their "weekend recreation."

After a career of listening to patient after remorseful patient telling me how they ruined their lives forever, pursuing what they thought was going to be fun, recreational, sporty or exciting, I'm struck by how much of the arthritis I see is at least in part self-inflicted. And since this is about the only aspect of OA that is truly preventable, I think we should wise up and start taking better care of our joints—and that means putting them less at risk.

Weight and Arthritis

Sporting foolishness aside, by far the most preventable joint damage is that inflicted by too much weight across a weight-bearing joint. When I see morbidly obese patients with sore knees and feet, I'm looking at evolution gone amuck. The knee, for instance, bears peak loads of about 5 times your body weight, so even at 200 pounds that's half a ton of compressive load. Go to the museum and look at a mammoth or any dinosaur. They had huge joints for their huge weight. We have little joints and then we load them with mammoth amounts of weight. Is it any wonder that the cartilage wears down?

"Is There a Diet for Arthritis?"

Patients ask me all the time what they should eat to help their arthritis. When I'm looking at an overweight patient on the exam table, I'm inclined to say, "Well, shall we start with what you *shouldn't* eat?" Clearly the most important nutritional contribution to keeping your joints healthy is keeping your weight at or near ideal weight for your frame and height. It is no wonder that all the insurance actuarial tables start with age, height, weight and go straight to smoking habits. The same is true for the health of your joints. You can't control the calendar, but you do have control over your weight. Sure, skinny people get arthritis too, but they tolerate it much better, they go longer before they need surgery and they do better if they finally need surgery.

The bookshelves are lined with claims for this diet or that nutritional supplement, this herb or that extract, which seem to have the magical powers to cure arthritis. The evidence presented in these books is usually anecdotal, the "studies", if there are any, are quasi-scientific, financed by the company selling the potion, and the results are literally too good to be true. The idea that swallowing shark cartilage or flax seeds or some new combination of vitamins will reverse damage to articular cartilage or even control the symptoms of osteoarthritis is a fairy tale, plain and simple. We're talking Peter Pan here, folks. If you close your eyes and wish hard enough, there really is a Never-Never-Land. If all these things worked, every orthopedist and rheumatologist in the world would be taking this stuff right now. But we're not. We're trying to make sense out of the latest P.T. Barnum barking on the midway of the Arthritis Circus.

The Arthritis Foundation, a leading organization in the study of joint diseases, says the following about unsubstantiated diet claims:

> *"Unproven Diet Claims*
> *Today, there are many claims that special diets, foods or supplements can cause or cure arthritis. Many of these claims generate a lot of publicity. The idea that there are simple answers to complicated autoimmune diseases is very appealing. Unfortunately, most claims for cure-all diets or nutritional supplements have not been scientifically tested to determine if they work and if they are safe. The scientific studies associated with these claims are often incomplete and may be harmful instead of beneficial.*
>
> *Some diets and supplements promoted as arthritis cures are outright frauds; others simply haven't been sufficiently tested. Some of the specific diets that are known to have harmful side effects include those that rely on large doses of alfalfa, copper salts or zinc, or the so-called immune power diet or the low-calorie/low-fat/low-protein diet."* [2]

2 http://www.arthritis.org/AFStore/StartRead.asp?idProduct=3358

44

Their suggestions for a healthy diet make no claims to cure arthritis, but are reasonable recommendations for anyone who wants to feel better generally.

Guidelines for a Healthy Diet*

- Eat a variety of foods, and avoid those that can interact with your medications.
- Maintain a healthy weight.
- Use fat and cholesterol in moderation.
- Eat plenty of vegetables, fruits and whole-grain products.
- Use sugar and salt in moderation.
- Drink alcohol in moderation.
- Take in the daily requirements of vitamins and minerals, including calcium[3].

Hard to disagree with any of that! But notice there are no specific recommendations for herbs and spices, extracts or emulsions. That's because none of that stuff works. OK?

Making Sense Out of Exercise for Arthritis

Exercise for arthritic joints should be divided into those exercises that are beneficial in preventing OA and maintaining healthy joints, as opposed to those exercises that will benefit an already arthritic joint. This may seem a subtle distinction, but in fact it's critical. Arthritic joints will simply not tolerate the same exercises that healthy, undamaged joints will enjoy.

Healthy joints need strengthening exercises for the muscles that motor them, stretching exercises to maintain flexibility and range of motion, and aerobic conditioning to resist fatigue which can lead to joint injury. Arthritic joints need

3   http://www.arthritis.org/AFStore/StartRead.asp?idProduct=3358

exercises that maintain and strengthen their muscles too, but without hurting the joint itself—adding insult to injury. These exercises also need to maintain the joint's compromised range of motion, but stretching can't be expected to restore or achieve a normal range of motion. Let's take the example of the normal versus the arthritic knee.

The normal knee is capable of lifting the body's weight against resistance—that's what it does climbing every stair—without batting an eye. It can sustain the impact of jogging, and the stress of deep knee bending and full knee extension, for stretching the muscles. So one could design a program that involved running, StairMaster, cycling—you name it. The arthritic knee could not tolerate jogging or probably stair climbing, yet may do fine with lower impact activities like cycling or swimming.

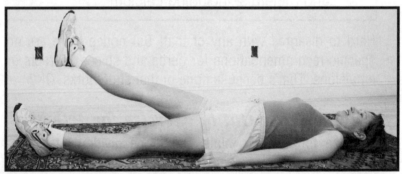

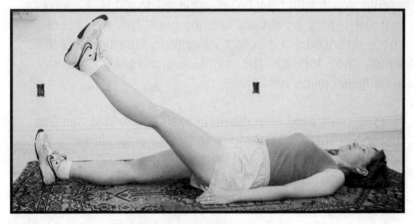

For sore joints, we commonly prescribe "isometric" exercises. These are exercises that involve simultaneously contracting the muscles that act as antagonists across a joint. For the knee that might mean contracting both the quadriceps and the hamstrings at the same time and lifting the leg up while lying down. In this way, all the muscles groups that cross the knee are exercised and strengthened without having to move the sore joint at all. You can apply the same principle to create an isometric exercise for the muscles that motor any joint—without stressing the arthritic joint.

For stretching sore joints, Tai Chi and yoga (kept within reason) may help arthritic patients maintain what flexibility the damaged joint can muster. It's important not to stress these worn out joints *beyond* their limited range of motion, as this may incite a pain response, muscle spasm and a vicious cycle of pain, spasm and more limitation. I'm particularly alarmed about some of the fanatical yoga exercises like Pilates. Here's their philosophy:

> Pilates' *"...unique teaching philosophy - the Core Connections anatomical paradigm of mapping and toning the body's vital fitness relationships - grounding through the bones, using length-tension muscle balance and breath as energy."* [4]

I'm a little nervous about anything "grounding through the bones." Again, I think almost any exercise is great for the healthy body—I'm talking about the arthritis sufferer here.

Pilate to your heart's content, if you don't hurt. But if you try to stretch a worn out joint, you only get pain and more pain.

4   http://www.pilatescenterofaustin.com/questions.html

What Can a Physical Therapist Do for Your Arthritis?

- PT's main role is to teach you what you can do for yourself.
- PT can teach you exercises to strengthen the muscles that support the joints.
- PT can teach you to maintain but usually not regain lost joint motion.
- PT can advise you what activities to avoid that will worsen your symptoms.
- PT can design an exercise program that is right for your arthritis.

Prescribing aerobic exercise for arthritic patients requires a little creativity also. Water aerobics are the absolute best for worn out joints, providing a supportive environment, and graduated resistance. But stationary cycling and even seated exercise with light weights in the hands can accomplish much the same goals. If this all sounds a little geriatric for you boomers out there, remember that professional athletes now use pool resistance training for both speed and aerobic exercise.

"So What Can You Do for Me, Doctor?"

Up to now, I've focused on what the therapists would call "arthritis self-help"—those things that the patient can and should do to live with arthritis. I've emphasized prevention, sensible exercise and education. Most patients listen respectfully while I lecture them on losing weight, getting on a reasonable exercise program and even while I lacerate their fanciful hopes of better joints through alfalfa. But eventually we get down to what people really come to me for: drugs and surgery.

Frontline Drugs in the Treatment of Osteoarthritis

The frontline drugs we use in alleviating at least some of the symptoms of OA are the non-narcotic analgesics (pain killers) like Tylenol (acetaminophen) and the so-called non-steroidal anti-inflammatory drugs or NSAIDs. Aspirin could be considered an NSAID but ibuprofen in all its aliases (Advil, Motrin, Nuprin, to name a few) is probably the one you're most familiar with. I've watched these drugs come and go—I remember when ibuprofen came out—and at any given point in time there are now something like twenty-five or thirty of them out there on the market: Clinoril (sulindac) , Relafen (nabumetone), Daypro (oxaprozin), Naprosyn (naproxen), Feldene (piroxicam)—I could go on. Some are available over-the-counter and some just by prescription. They all share the same effects and side effects. The upside is they work both as analgesics to relieve joint pain and as anti-inflammatories to relieve some of the joint swelling. Neither of these two types of medication really gets at the heart of the process that is OA. Neither does insulin take away your diabetes or Claritin (loratadine) your allergies. But they are helpful for symptomatic relief, or at least control. Sometimes they seem like wonder drugs; sometimes they seem more like sugar pills. Some people can take them for years without so much as a belch; others take a couple and their stomach falls out. Most of the side effects are self-limiting and involve upsetting the digestive system or causing easy bruising or bleeding. But there is a significant incidence of gastrointestinal bleeding and ulcers when taken regularly in therapeutic doses. In a few patients, there are long-term effects on the kidney. Like any drug, true allergies can occur, in which case the symptoms are dramatic and usually sudden.

The Life Cycle of the Latest Wonder Drug

Eventually, almost every new NSAID goes through a life-cycle, driven by the symbiotic fantasies of the poor suffering patients who want the pill that's finally going to "cure" arthritis, and by the avarice of the parent drug company that wants to make gazillions of dollars off those same poor suffering patients. If this seems a little cynical, trust me, I have watched these drugs come and go over the past 25 years. They have a life cycle that goes something like this.

Every new drug is a wonder drug with few side effects. It's always "more effective" and "easier on the stomach" than the current best drug—and more expensive. Each one comes in prettier packaging with a cute, clever name and more hype than the last one. The drug peddlers come to the doctors' offices passing out free lunches and ballpoint pens with outrageous, memorable color schemes, and the race is on. Some has-been celebrity athlete appears on television saying that this drug helped him to shoot par on the back nine, when only a week before he was in a wheelchair. Patients start coming in asking for the new wonder drug and wondering why it's not on their insurance plan's formulary yet. In this sense, all patients seem remnants of the 60's: "Hell, if there's a better drug out there, why can't I have it *now*?"

So, we doctors try the drug, pass out a few samples and sit back to see if it's any different from every other NSAID that's ever come out. Inevitably, after a few months, the hype settles down, a few reports of fatal liver failure or dramatic allergic reaction come out and are overblown by the media. Patients, who were on it for a while, report that it really isn't that different than the wonder drug they were on last year. The colorful ballpoint pens run out of ink, the cost of the pill slowly comes down from the ionosphere and the latest greatest cure for arthritis becomes just another box of samples on the shelf.

A few really effective new drugs did come out, and then had to be taken off the market due to a truly scary incidence of side effects. In fact, when I see a drug that seems to actually work better than all its peers, I assume that it's going to be off the market in a few months and usually curtail my use, waiting for those most reliable of medical journals, *60 Minutes* and *20/20,* to tell us the real scoop. By the time Mike Wallace and Barbara Walters are lambasting it, you better have stopped prescribing it.

So that's the way this business operates. By the time any NSAID comes out, there is so much invested in it, that the companies just have to push it with all they've got. Unfortunately, if the drug doesn't live up to its expectations, the patients are the ones who suffer. There are a lot of relatively safe and effective NSAIDs out there, but none is the cure for arthritis and, at the level of the joint, none is better, cheaper or more flexible than ibuprofen. That's what I take for my arthritis.

Hot Off the Presses: the COX-2 Inhibitors

A new class of drugs has come out recently that is worth discussing, not because they seem to be any better at alleviating the symptoms of arthritis, but because they may be easier on the stomach. These are the so-called COX-2 inhibitors. Of course, these are being promoted as the "super drugs" for arthritis. The pharmacology of these is slightly different than the traditional NSAIDs in that they have less of an effect on the stomach lining—at least in theory. So far, there are three main drugs in this category, Celebrex (celexobid), Vioxx (rofecoxib) and Bextra (valdecoxib).

Celebrex is a good drug. In my practice, Vioxx seems to be a better analgesic, but I see side effects more commonly. But remember: it's not that these COX-2 inhibitors are better in treating the symptoms of arthritis; the advance is that they are significantly less risky to take because the stomach more easily tolerates them. Even then, there are still some patients who get gastrointestinal problems with these drugs too. Right now the COX-2 drugs are at the peak of the life cycle I was talking about.

The latest controversy is that these drugs may not have as much effect in preventing heart attack, as some of the older NSAIDs. This has been picked up in the press and serves as a great example of lay people misinterpreting scientific data. These drugs were *never designed to have any effect on heart disease*, but the older NSAIDs did thin the blood more. OK, that's either a bothersome side effect (easy bruising, bleeding complications with surgery) or it's a benefit (acts like aspirin to prevent the clots in the coronary arteries that can cause heart attacks), depending on your point of view. Either way it has little to do with what the drug is actually supposed to do. Along come the COX-2 drugs and they possess fewer of these blood thinning side effects, which can then be seen as a blessing (fewer bleeding complications at surgery, fewer bleeding ulcers, etc.) or a curse (lower rate of protection against heart attacks) when compared to the older drugs. By the time this rather predictable observation comes out on the evening news, the talking heads have us thinking that these new drugs cause heart attacks, or at least don't prevent them as well as the older drugs which are never prescribed to prevent heart attacks anyway. (The FDA requires the label of Vioxx to say that while the arthritis drug causes fewer ulcers, it may increase the risk of heart attack. Taking one coated baby aspirin a day can neutralize this risk.) Vioxx has been associated with at least seven cases of aseptic meningitis, inflammation of the spinal fluid, as of this writing. Other anti-inflammatories including those you can buy over-the-counter may cause aseptic meningitis also. As I said above, all anti-inflammatory arthritis medicines have the potential for toxicity to the stomach and kidneys, more common than this rare side-effect of meningitis, but people must weigh the risks and benefits.

Doctors presently do not use long term Vioxx, Celebrex or Bextra in those with failing kidneys and failing hearts. We tend not to use Vioxx in patients who develop the side effect of swollen ankles or in patients with known coronary artery disease, just in case there is something to the concern about causing heart attacks in those predisposed. We are cautious about using these drugs in asthmatics if they have a history of aspirin sensitivity as some asthmatics do. Celebrex should not be prescribed to those with a sulfa allergy.

Currently, I have to say that my jury is out on the COX-2 inhibitors. They are still under study and, though prescribed widely (Celebrex is already one of the most widely prescribed drugs in the world), I'd say they too are in that early part of the NSAID marketing life cycle where all is rosy, hopeful, and expensive. The ballpoint pens haven't run out yet, and maybe they won't. But don't get your hopes up for a drug to cure arthritis. In fairness, their pharmaceutical companies do not make that claim, but you sure wouldn't know it listening to the joyous commercials on the evening news.

Celebrate! Celebrate!
Dance to the Music!
Have a pill!
Pay the bill!
Dance to the Music!

Glucosamine, Chondroitin and Other Supplements

These medications represent another area in which we don't know yet where we're going. The latest drug group getting attention for arthritis treatment is the glucosamine and chondroitin preparations. These are being called "chondro-protective" agents, or literally "cartilage protecting" drugs. These are actually sold as nutritional supplements and are not considered drugs by the FDA, but that could change. They are readily available over-the-counter in the vitamin and nutritional supplement corner of your local drugstore, and nobody really knows whether they work or how they do, if indeed they do. They claim to "Regenerate, Rebuild and Renew!" your joints. In other words, the hope is that they can actually heal the damaged articular cartilage in OA.

There have been a limited number of studies of these drugs both in this country and in Europe. Both these molecules (chondroitin and glucosamine) are parts of the complex building blocks that make up the matrix of articular cartilage. By matrix, I mean the substance that gives cartilage its shock absorbing quality—the stuff that fills in the gaps between beams and joists of collagen fibers. The assumption is that when you swallow these molecules in large doses, they somehow get into your joints and help repair the damage that we call osteoarthritis. This is an attractive concept, but I'm not sure it makes sense physiologically. I have a hard time understanding how these large macromolecules could get through the digestive tract (unchanged), into the blood stream (unmolested), then into the joint fluid and, finally, be taken up into the articular cartilage. Even if this is physiologically possible, there is no evidence that articular cartilage has ever been healed in this way. The real problem with all the studies on these drugs in this country is that they have been too short—usually no more than three months—to fairly judge either the effects or the potential side effects.

So as a scientist I'm trained to be skeptical. Perhaps there is something beneficial that we don't quite understand yet. I have lots of patients who have come into the office telling me that they've started taking this stuff and they feel better. Some have been able to stop taking their NSAIDs after a few months on glucosamine. The orthopedic and rheumatology communities are keeping an open mind on these drugs. So far the American College of Rheumatology, the American Academy of Orthopedic Surgeons and the Arthritis Foundation all believe it is premature to endorse the use of these agents. But unlike the fad diets and herbal supplements, many arthritic orthopods and rheumatologists take this stuff themselves. There are larger clinical trials going on as we speak that may help define the role of these agents. These studies should be out in the next year or two.

In the Meantime, Should We Recommend Chondroitin and Glucosamine?

Here's what I tell my patients. First, I don't know exactly how these drugs work, but they probably can't really "rebuild" or "regenerate" anything, so don't come back in three months expecting to see your x-ray looking better. They may have a protective effect on the already arthritic joint, and I haven't seen any side effects at all from taking these preparations, so there seems to be little downside risk, other than weight loss in your wallet. If you're going to try one of them, take it for at least a month and don't change your other arthritis regimen at the same time. Make just this one change, and we'll see what happens. If you feel better at the end of that month, keep taking the drug. I think that's a rational way to approach any new drug, but remember: we could find out next month that it causes death by flatulence, so keep an open mind.

"Can't You Just Cut Out This Pain, Doctor?"

The surgery for arthritic joints is almost always salvage surgery for a joint irrevocably damaged. As I said earlier, we don't have many things we can do that truly reverse the process of osteoarthritis. Now that you understand that OA is organ failure in that organ we call the joint, this makes a little more sense. No one does a heart transplant for anything but a hopelessly failed heart and I don't do knee replacements unless the knee is shot. But this hasn't kept surgeons from trying to find operations that will arrest or reverse the damage of osteoarthritis. Most of what we do surgically boils down to trying to prevent or delay the onset of OA—by skillfully fixing joint fractures, for instance—or replacing the completely worn out joint with a prosthesis or artificial joint. Total joint replacement is one of the miraculous surgical developments of the 20th century. It restores patients to pain-free walking with a low complication rate and remarkable durability. We now expect at least 90% of our implants to survive 10 years or more. I'm going to discuss the evolution and current state of total joint replacement shortly, but before that, I need to explain to you the "paradigm of arthroplasty."

The Paradigm of Arthroplasty

Nowadays everything has a paradigm or worse yet, a "paradigm shift." But I've been teaching this one to my residents for 20 years, so this is not the new, sexy kind of paradigm. This is an old-fashioned way of thinking about surgery for arthritis. "Arthro-plasty" means "to change the joint", and in general refers to any operation designed to realign, reconstruct or replace a worn out joint.

Before hip replacement was pioneered in the 1960s, what an orthopedic surgeon could do to an arthritic joint was limited. If it was crooked, he could realign it by cutting the bones above or below it. This is called an "osteotomy." If it was a smaller joint whose motion was expendable, he could fuse it. Our term for this is "arthrodesis." He could cut the bad joint out and let it fill in with scar tissue. This is called a "resection" arthroplasty. He could cut it out and borrow something from the neighboring tissues to act as a spacer—stuff in some nearby tendon, say. This would be a "resection, interposition" arthroplasty. Finally, as techniques and metallurgy advanced, he could cut it out, and replace one side of the joint with a metal prosthesis that mimicked the missing joint surface. This was called an "endoprosthesis."

Now as crazy as those alternatives may sound to you, we still use every one of them today for some joint, in some cases. We still do osteotomies around the knee. We fuse small joints in the fingers and toes frequently. We do resection interposition arthroplasties for arthritis at the base of the thumb and sometimes the bunion joint. And we do endoprostheses for broken hips and shoulders all the time. The paradigm is this: for any arthritic joint, the surgeon must think through all the available options—essentially in their historical order of appearance—before deciding what the best option for that joint is. Though joint replacements have been miraculous for the hip, knee and shoulder, they have had only limited success in the elbow, and ankle and have been downright lousy in the wrist, and most small joints of the hands and feet. This may change, but I'll start with the overwhelming success story: hip replacement.

The Success Story: Total Hip Replacement
When it comes to arthritis surgery, everything changed with

the development of hip joint replacement. Total hip replacement is still one of the most amazing operations we have. It has revolutionized orthopedics, and we owe it all to one guy: Dr. John Charnley. In the 1960s, after a career that would have made him famous for several other major contributions to the specialty, this quiet little perfectionist, operating in near obscurity in Lancashire County, England, changed the lives of millions of people. He literally invented all the major aspects of total joint replacement, as we know it today. He invented the metal on plastic prosthesis, the cement that keeps it in place, the laminar flow (ultra-clean) operating rooms we use, the total body exhaust or "space suits" that we wear doing this and most other joint replacements. He pioneered all these innovations, working at the Wrightington Center for Hip Surgery, formally a hospital for surgical tuberculosis patients, almost in the middle of nowhere. Charnley persisted through early failures and gave us an operation that is done over 250,000 times every year in this country alone. All those surgeons who brought this procedure to the United States, including my mentor Dr. Mark Coventry at the Mayo Clinic, had to make the pilgrimage to Wrightington to learn the procedure from Charnley. In no small way, every one of us who does this operation is a descendent of this great man, so forgive me if I slip from admiration to reverence when I say he's my hero.

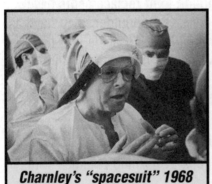

Charnley's "spacesuit" 1968

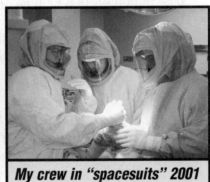

My crew in "spacesuits" 2001

Total hip replacement is an operation originally designed for older patients with severe arthritis of the hip. Because nothing implanted in the human body can last forever, the decision to have a hip replaced in the boomer age

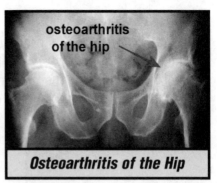

Osteoarthritis of the Hip

group is still a big one. The elderly patient is not likely to outlive his prosthesis, but the boomer almost certainly is. Before he considers it, the patient should make sure he is committed to accepting the risks of surgery and the rigors of the rehab. He should be sure that he has come to the end of his rope, tied a knot and fallen off. If it seems to be a hard decision, you probably don't really need it yet. Your hip will let you know when it's time. It all boils down to the Big Question, "Is this bothering you enough to have a big operation to fix it?" If the answer comes back, "I don't know...", then don't have surgery.

Total hip replacement involves replacing the worn out socket with a metal and plastic one,

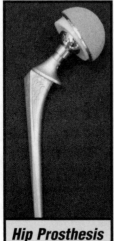

...and replacing the worn out femoral head with a metal ball that fits into the plastic socket. In other words, the procedure is a metal-on-plastic ball and socket replacement of a biological ball and socket joint.

The surgery takes about one and a half to two

Hip Prosthesis   **Hip Replacement**

hours. The recovery is prompt and most patients are free of their hip pain right away. But there are limitations, and these restrictions hit the boomer generation much harder. You can't jump or twist too much or run or bend too much with a hip replacement.

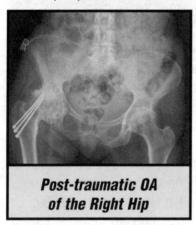

Post-traumatic OA of the Right Hip

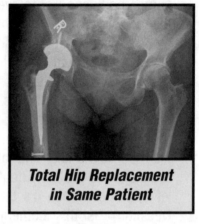

Total Hip Replacement in Same Patient

The life expectancy of these prostheses is in the neighborhood of ten to fifteen years, so you do the math. Emily has her hip replacement at thirty-five and at the ripe old age of fifty she's looking at her first hip revision. Revising a worn out artificial joint is a lot harder than it sounds. The bone is weaker than the first go-around, the old parts may not want to come out, the soft tissues are getting scarred and the muscles are getting beat up. Revisions are hard cases with a higher complication rate than primary hip replacement. But, in spite of the cold facts, some patients have little choice. If a hip is completely worn out from one of several childhood hip diseases, or simply from early osteoarthritis, a hip replacement in the middle years is inevitable. Once you've had it, a few activities are out, but at least you can walk without pain. I will go into more detail on the specifics of hip replacement in *"Chapter 9: The Hip"*.

The evolution of knee replacement lagged behind hip replacement by about a decade. It didn't become a consistently successful operation until the late 1970s. But since then, knee replacement has become every bit as miraculous as hip replacement. The number of knee replacements done yearly in the US now exceeds hip replacement. At

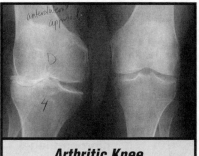

Arthritic Knee

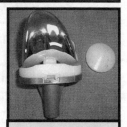

Prosthetic Knee

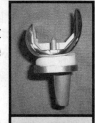

Prosthetic Knee

our institution it is not uncommon to replace both knees at the same operation—as radical as that sounds. I will touch more on the specifics of knee, and shoulder replacement surgery in their respective chapters (Chapters 10 and 4).

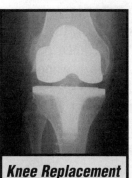

Knee Replacement

Worn-out Cartilage

But what about surgery for the joint before it has failed? Can anything be done in the early or middle stages of arthritis to buy a little time? I'll use the knee as an example for this discussion.

In the knee, the first thing that starts to wear out is often the meniscus—that little semi-lunar piece of gristle that sits between the two big bones of the knee, the femur above and the tibia below. The menisci are unique to the knee and have several functions, but for these purposes, it will suffice to think of them as rubbery washers that share the load in the joint.

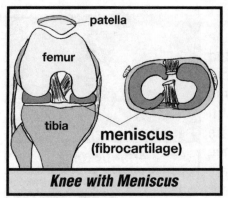

Knee with Meniscus

patella

femur

tibia

meniscus (fibrocartilage)

The one on the inner side of the joint, which we call the medial meniscus, usually wears out first, and usually in the back of the knee before the front. The result is some combination of pain along the inner (medial) side of the knee, swelling, catching and an overall feeling that something is not right. This condition is so common that it is usually diagnosed by the history, physical exam and plain x-rays. Though we sometimes get an MRI, it is just as likely that we won't. If a guy my age comes in with medial knee pain, tenderness along the joint line on that side, a little swelling in the knee, a catch when I stress his knee the right way and normal X-rays, well, he's got a degenerative tear of the medial meniscus and we scope his knee.

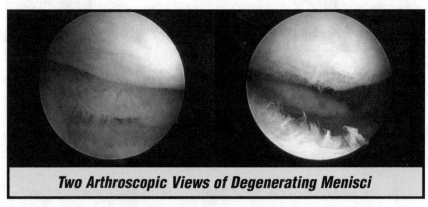

Two Arthroscopic Views of Degenerating Menisci

By "scope," I mean that we usually treat this condition with arthroscopic removal of the torn part of the cartilage. And though the patient will get significant improvement and his knee will usually even act like a normal joint for some years to come, in fact, it is not a normal knee. It's a knee in the early phases of osteoarthritis and the owner should modify his physical activities to minimize risky behaviors, such as sports that require a lot of stopping, starting and twisting, or load the joint with impact (jogging). He should also get to know his surgeon, because they are about to develop a long-term relationship.

Hear now the "Parable of the Laborer and the Lawyer." This illustrates who can be helped by arthroscopic surgery and who might not be. Two forty-something patients presented to the orthopedic surgeon. Both had medial knee pain. One was a maintenance supervisor for a public school. He had a high school education and his job involved heavy lifting, squatting, climbing and kneeling. The other was a corporate lawyer whose physical activities included heavy drinking, hot sex and vigorous litigation. The laborer had constant aching pain, mild swelling, no mechanical symptoms, and a standing knee x-ray that showed mild medial joint space narrowing. The lawyer had a localized catching on the medial side of his knee, intermittent symptoms and a pristine looking x-ray.

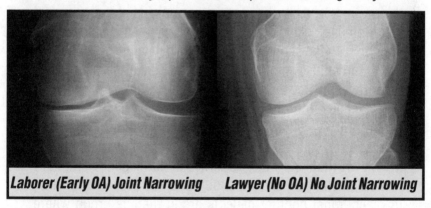

Laborer (Early OA) Joint Narrowing   **Lawyer (No OA) No Joint Narrowing**

Both patients had arthroscopic surgery but one didn't get better. Why? The answer is easy: the laborer already had arthritis and the lawyer just had a torn meniscus. Arthroscopy can't do much for arthritis. You can't put back articular cartilage. If the x-ray shows that the cartilage is wearing out, I know that when I look inside that knee with the scope that it will be like opening a coffin to look at a dead man—and just about as effective. The lawyer gets his torn meniscus nibbled out and lives to prosecute another day. The laborer is still limping back to the office two months later, asking questions about disability, cursing his surgeon for not helping him and cursing himself for not going to college. The smart surgeon would have discouraged the laborer from having arthroscopic surgery for his arthritic knee.

Recently, a well-designed and controlled study compared arthroscopic knee surgery for the arthritic knee to a sham surgery where nothing was actually done. The outcomes were the same. Patients with the "placebo surgery" showed just as much improvement as those who underwent arthroscopic "washouts" or debridements. For years, most good orthopedists have known this. It makes sense. You can't really repair any cartilage damage with the arthroscope—at least not in the arthritic knee. You can cut things out and if the patient complains of mechanical symptoms—locking, catching, giving way—it is still justified to go in with the scope and take out whatever is catching. But don't be deluded into thinking that will take the pain of the arthritic joint away. You can't cut out pain with an arthroscope. Prior to arthroscopic surgery in the boomer patient, I try very hard to explain that if I find torn meniscus cartilage and can tidy that up, he may get some relief. If I find mostly arthritis and worn out articular cartilage, I won't have helped much at all, and we should both be prepared for that. In reality most boomer patients are in the age group where we first see meniscal degeneration and where the articular cartilage damage is minor. I have more trouble explaining to the 75 year-old patient with frank osteoarthritis on his x-ray that scoping his knee will not help at all.

Summary of Surgery for OA

Though we have a culture of high hopes and even higher expectations, it is important to hammer home this point: we still have no surgical treatments that reverse the process of osteoarthritis. We have some very successful salvage operations—transplants really—for the end stage hip, knee and shoulder. In the early stages of knee degeneration, there is an indication for arthroscopically trimming out the worn out meniscus, if it is producing mechanical symptoms or pain. And for almost every joint there is some procedure within our paradigm of arthroplasty that can be applied: small joints can be fused; some joints do well with osteotomies or resection-interposition arthroplasties. Within each individual section of this book, I will discuss all the operations for arthritis, as they apply to that specific joint.

The Other Kind of Arthritis: Rheumatoid Arthritis (RA)

Unlike its common cousin, osteoarthritis (OA), rheumatoid arthritis (RA) is a less common but more devastating disease. OA affects mainly the weight-bearing joints and certain hardworking joints in the hands. Since this condition becomes more common with age, after fifty or sixty almost everyone has it in some joint, if only to a minor degree. RA on the other hand may occur at any age from infancy to old age, and spares no joint, large or small. Worse yet, in its most flagrant form, it may affect the kidneys, the skin and even the salivary glands. I'll be discussing the effect it has on the joints, but it is critical to understand that RA is a disease of the whole body with the worst manifestations seen in the joints.

RA usually has a rather sudden onset. I've had patients who can tell me the day, and even the hour when their life

65

changed. It can be more insidious than that, but for many patients, it has a very discrete starting point. RA is what we call an "auto-immune" disease. By that we mean that, for some reason, the body begins to act as if it is allergic to itself. The actual stimulus for this phenomenon is still unknown, but suddenly the body's immune system gets misdirected towards its own joints. The powerful cells and

Clues That Your Arthritis May Be More Than Just OA

- Multiple joints involved all at once
- Dramatic morning stiffness lasting hours
- Symptoms outside the joints: malaise, fever, rash
- Lack of response to over-the-counter medicines

chemicals usually responsible for ridding the body of invaders and foreigners, attack the joint's soft tissue lining—remember the synovium?—and literally try to digest it, as if the body were somehow trying to eat its own joints. The inflammation that arises from this process typically involves severe swelling, warmth, pain and stiffness in many joints at once. There may be associated fever and other symptoms that give a clue that this is a *systemic* disease, and not simple osteoarthritis.

Destruction by Friendly Fire

One way to look at the cellular events that cause the disease we call rheumatoid arthritis is to use the analogy of a tank battle. In this battle, the "friendly" tanks are the immune cells that usually defend the joint from invasion by foreign or "hostile" tanks. When things go right, these "friendlies" detect the invading hostile forces at some distance to the joint, communicate with each other, and then together they advance and attack the hostiles, dispatching them and protecting the joint. An example of a hostile force might be some bacteria introduced near the joint through a puncture wound. The friendly tanks mass around this invading force and blow it away with their various weapon systems. But critical to the success of this operation is the ability to accurately discriminate between friend and foe. What happens in RA is that some as yet unknown trigger tricks the friendly tanks into mistaking their own forces for attackers. The friendly tanks begin firing on their colleagues, and the joint is destroyed in the crossfire by what the military so poignantly calls, "Friendly Fire."

In the early stages the treatment of RA mainly involves making the right diagnosis, discriminating it from other systemic diseases that may involve the joints, and then treating it aggressively with drugs that suppress the immune system and the inflammation that is the hallmark of the disease. This is usually done by internists and sometimes by a particular internal medicine specialist called a "rheumatologist." But often, since it's a joint problem, the patient may go to the orthopedist first. This can make for a tricky diagnosis, especially if the disease is early or just presenting in one or only a few joints. Luckily there are several blood tests that can help. These include general tests of inflammation and also a specific test that looks for the disease's effect on the immune system, the rheumatoid factor. Though not all patients with RA have a positive rheumatoid factor—especially cases of childhood RA—when this factor is positive, it is quite helpful in the diagnosis. These same blood tests are universally negative in OA.

Preventing the Damage from "Friendly Fire"

The drug treatment of RA is evolving. Recently rheumatologists have become more aggressive, using medicines that are almost like the chemotherapeutic agents used in treating cancer. However, they usually start with many of the same simple anti-inflammatory drugs that we use in OA. When these are not effective, they accelerate the treatment to drugs like cortisone and gold shots. Gold salts have been used in the treatment of RA for hundreds of years and now are given as weekly intramuscular injections. This can cause temporary remission of the disease but usually can't be continued longer than two years because of toxicity. Other big guns like methotrexate, a drug used in cancer chemotherapy, are also used to suppress the immune system in an attempt to arrest the disease process.

An exciting new development is drugs designed to work against one of the specific communication links in the friendly fire chain of command and control. Imagine that during a battle involving friendly fire (the auto-immune process), the friendly tanks could be blinded by blocking the orders to fire that are coming from their central command post. Without orders to keep firing, they would cease firing and, in the process, stop destroying their own troops. This is exactly what the two new drugs, Remicaide (infliximab) and Enbrel (etanercept) do. These are smart weapons targeted against the command bunker that is issuing the faulty orders against the joints by their own friendly forces. By blocking the signals to the immune response, it gets at the very heart of the problem in RA. As with all new drugs, time will tell if this is the major advance it seems to be in the laboratory.

RA is often called the "crippling" arthritis, but it might better be called the "deforming" arthritis since OA of the hip or knee can be equally crippling. RA can ravage any joint, but when it gangs up on the hands and feet, it can leave them devastated. RA is the second most common reason for the three big joint replacements that I do: hip, knee and shoulder. But it is the number one reason for the more unusual joint replacements we do: elbow and ankle. Luckily, RA patients often do quite well with joint replacements, but they are higher risk patients. This is due to the medicines they are usually taking and the way those medicines suppress the immune system, and to the general debilitating nature of the disease itself. Infections and other soft-tissue healing problems are much more common in rheumatoid patients. Rheumatoid skin can become so fragile that it actually tears while manipulating a fracture or even positioning a patient for surgery.

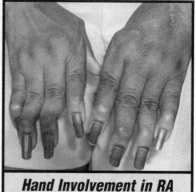

Hand Involvement in RA

Rheumatoid arthritis is more manageable with the modern drugs and some of our joint replacement operations, but it still ranks first among the systemic diseases that I wouldn't wish on my worst enemy.

Are We Going to Cure Arthritis in Our Lifetime?

The short answer is "don't count on it." In fact, I'd say we're more likely to find a cure for rheumatoid arthritis—which probably has some one antecedent stimulus that sets the immune system attacking itself—than we are to find a cure for osteoarthritis, which has so many heterogeneous causes. New drugs will come out that may be more effective at controlling certain aspects of the symptoms, but like all drugs, they'll have their own life-cycle. There will be new pens for my pocket, new ads on TV and billions of dollars will change hands, but in the end, joints will keep failing because human joints are woefully under-designed. They are not designed to stand up to a population that's overweight, overworked and living well beyond the original date of obsolescence. Though it has been around forever—osteoarthritis has been found in the hips of Neanderthals, cave bears and Egyptian mummies—it wasn't such a big deal when people only lived into their fourth decade and competed with the sabertooth tigers for food.

What advances do come in the treatment of osteoarthritis will come from genuine scientific research and be confirmed by well-controlled studies in large populations of patients. That goes for surgery as well as medical remedies. If someone suggests to you that they've found the "cure" for arthritis or even a new dazzling treatment, be it herbal, medical or surgical, ask to see the data. Don't be suckered by anecdotes, testimonials or three-minute "focus" reports on the evening news. In the next few chapters I will discuss region by region, what happens as your musculoskeletal system advances along with you into your middle years. I assume you want the facts and not just the fantasies.

Chapter 4: The Shoulder

This is a subject that is very personal for me since I've had a chronic rotator cuff problem in my right shoulder for years. The common problems I see with the shoulder include a host of issues and injuries related to the rotator cuff muscles, shoulder dislocations, true arthritis of the shoulder and its adjacent supporting joints, and, finally, fractures of the shoulder. I'm going to focus on those specific conditions that afflict the midlife population that visits me everyday in my clinic.

The large number of patients my age I see with sore shoulders is second only to those with bum knees. The shoulder is another great example of either God's great handiwork or his sloppy design, depending on your spin on things. The purpose of the shoulder is to allow us to put our hand anywhere in space we want to put it. Among the major joints, it has the most remarkable range of motion. Compared to its other ball-and-socket joint cousin, the sturdy, weight-bearing hip, it's a world traveler. Most of us can reach to our opposite shoulder blade with our hand, both from the front over the other shoulder and from behind the back. Try something like that with your foot and you'll appreciate the shoulder's incredible adaptation for movement.

But what it boasts in mobility, it also lacks in stability. It is by far the easiest major joint to dislocate or to put out of joint. In fact, it is held together with no bony stability at all. By this I mean the geometry of the shoulder joint has no reason to stay together and every reason to fall apart. Contrast it with the hip, which has a deep socket with the ball completely constrained within the socket. You can cut away all the muscles and ligaments (the straps that go from bone to bone across a joint to hold it together), and you will still have to exert a significant force to dislocate the hip. I have to do this every time we do a total hip replacement. Believe me, the hip is an inherently stable joint, and you would expect it to be, designed as it is for walking. On the other hand, the shoulder is a big round ball held up against a very shallow socket. It is held together not by the bony design, but by the ligaments and the muscles. And in the end it's those muscles that show the wear and tear. Collectively, we call these muscles the rotator cuff.

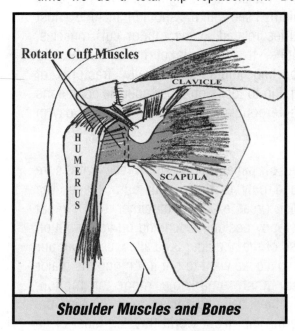

Shoulder Muscles and Bones

The healthy shoulder is a song sung in harmony among three sets of muscles.

The small rotator cuff muscles (the sopranos) begin mostly on the shoulder blade and attach around the ball (what surgeons call the "head") of the humerus. On their way from shoulder blade to shoulder, they pass under the over-arching end of the shoulder blade where the collarbone attaches. The collective job of these muscles is to direct the humeral head into the socket, so that the big, famous, glamorous muscles

72

(the tenors), the ones that you work out in the gym, can lift the arm or place the hand in space wherever necessary. These tenors have famous stage names like "the Delts" and "the Pecs" and "the Lats" (the deltoid, the pectorals, the latissimus dorsi). Finally, everyone knows you can't have a chorus without the basses. In this case, a third set of muscles helps position the shoulder blade on the chest. These muscles (the basses) we call the "scapular stabilizers," the scapula being our alias for the shoulder blade. The basses anchor the whole shoulder complex to the axial skeleton.

When these muscles groups work in harmony, doing those things that human beings are actually designed to do, the shoulder is truly a thing of beauty. But we boomers would be satisfied if the shoulder, like most of the body's wonders, just got on with its job.

Rotator Cuff Problems

The song goes sour when these muscles either get out of shape (deconditioning), get over used ("Honey, let's buy that Bowflex!"), or are asked to do what no shoulder should be asked to do ("Six games of racquetball and I whipped his butt!"). Each of the syndromes I described can have its damaging effect on the shoulder. The deconditioned may get tendonitis; the risk-taker may sustain a fracture; and the Narcissus or the aging jock may over-use the whole shoulder complex to the point where either the bones or the muscles are seriously injured.

The complaints are usually pain in the shoulder that worsens when we engage in overhead activities, almost always pain at night, various patterns of referred pain down the arm and dysfunction when using the shoulder. With the shoulder muscles, the underlying problem is almost always more functional than structural, and the solution is almost always more conservative than surgical.

Often, the rotator cuff muscles become tired or worn and, therefore, inefficient at doing their job, which, you recall, is to center the ball in the socket. Try as they might, the little sopranos get to where they can no longer balance the strong, overpowering, opera star tenors. The result is a condition we call "impingement." In this condition the rotator cuff muscles are overpowered by the lifting or throwing muscles, and the humeral head bangs into the roof over its head, resulting in pain and inflammation. The treatment is directed at avoiding the activities that aggravate the condition, using anti-inflammatory medications, sometimes injections of cortisone, and, most importantly, gradual, gentle rehabilitation of the rotator cuff muscles. Send the sopranos to rehab! That's the idea.

Just yesterday I saw a fellow boomer in the clinic with shoulder pain. He was actually an energetic guy working three jobs. He's had mild pain in his shoulder for a few years but never had to see the doctor about it before. When he gave me his history, I discovered that after many years of mild aggravation, his shoulder had recently gotten worse. He'd done some digging in the yard, which normally shouldn't have affected him that way because, believe me, his day job involves some heavy lifting. Other than that, he didn't recall any specific injury or incident. He experienced the pain over the outside of his shoulder, and it radiated down his arm to about where a short-sleeved shirt would end. It was worse with overhead activities and was giving him some real trouble sleeping. He didn't have any numbness in his hands or associated neck pain.

The physical exam revealed a full range of motion with pain at the extremes of flexion and rotation, and when I applied certain provocative maneuvers that are designed to specifically stress the muscles of the rotator cuff. ("Does it hurt when I do THISSSS?"). His strength was normal and the rest of the exam ruled out other causes. The x-rays were also normal.

He had a classic presentation of rotator cuff tendonitis, inflammation of and pain in the attachment of the sopranos into the humeral head. Though this is often called "Impingement Syndrome," that term is deceptively mechanical, implying that there is some abnormal anatomic arrangement that should be remedied surgically. In fact, this is the opening stanza in that symphony of gradual wear and tear on the cuff muscles. As I often tell patients, "This is what your mama would have called bursitis." Though that little sack that lies between the cuff tendon and the overlying bone—the bursa—does get inflamed, we now know that it is not the primary cause of the problem. Once the pain starts, the muscle gets weak and becomes increasingly inefficient in doing its job—centering the ball in the socket. The ball rides up as the tenors overpower the sopranos and the tendon impinges on the bone, which overhangs the shoulder.

The treatment for this is first to decrease the inflammation either by anti-inflammatory medicines taken by mouth or by the direct injection of cortisone into the area. But this is rarely the end of the problem and most patients will benefit from instruction in the exercises that can rehabilitate the weakened rotator cuff. In this case I gave him the injection and asked him to see the therapist in a week or so after some of the pain had calmed down.

Exercises are very easy to prescribe and not as easy to find the time to actually do. I spend a good deal of time trying to convince boomers who want that quick fix that their problem can be improved by a little regular exercise. The most willing patients, however, are usually those who really want to avoid surgery, or are suspicious that it's been offered too quickly. This describes a friend I treated who manages some of our investments. It's no secret that they don't teach financial management in medical school and that doctors are classically money "mis-managers". When Kathy and I first started to get a little cash built up, we hired a very knowledgeable financial manager, a guy with a Ph.D. and a way with mutual funds. This was pretty progressive thinking in the early 1980s. He lives in Los Angeles and has followed us as we transitioned from small-town Iowa, to San Antonio, and, finally, to New Orleans.

He developed chronic impingement syndrome and had seen several orthopedists. He had taken all the medicines and shots, but just wasn't getting better. His doctors were considering surgery. When he asked me about it, I described the shoulder mechanics and recommended the exercises that we do for chronic rotator cuff tendonitis. Here was an intelligent guy who only needed to understand the way the shoulder actually worked. He religiously did the therapy and, as expected, his symptoms resolved and have remained in abeyance for many years.

A more severe variant of this condition occurs when calcium deposits in the inflamed tendon. This is called "acute calcific tendonitis," with the emphasis on acute. Here the pain is more sudden and severe. I can certainly vouch for that—I had this problem once when I was about thirty-eight years old. I had recently started a weight-training program with some of my residents, all of them ten years younger than I was. They had me doing these presses with a barbell held behind the neck and then brought from that position to overhead and back. It felt great while I was doing it, but two days later I woke in the middle of the night with what felt like an ice pick sticking in my right shoulder. I couldn't lift my arm, and couldn't find a comfortable place to even rest it. The urgency of this problem was cranked up a notch by the fact that this was an operating day for me and I had three big cases to do, hip replacements and things like that. I got on the phone at 5:00 in the morning and called one of my fellow orthopods and said, "Man, you gotta meet me at the clinic and inject my shoulder so I can make it through the surgical list today." He obliged, meeting me at 6:30 and injecting my shoulder with cortisone. I had almost instant relief. I would have canceled the surgery, if I hadn't felt completely relieved. It felt like Androcles taking the thorn out of the lion's paw. Later after surgery, I stopped and got an x-ray that showed the calcium deposit in my tendon.

After this episode, I continued to have intermittent nagging pain off and on for the next ten years. It was never bad enough to keep me from doing anything I needed to do, but it bothered me, especially when I had to hold my hands out over the scrub sink for the five-minute wash-up before surgery. When I did the exercises that I hounded all my patients to do, guess what? I got better. When I'd get lax, the pain would creep back up on me. For the last several years I've been religious about my exercise program and I have no pain at all.

And that's the lesson here. This condition is often treated best with persistent exercises to strengthen the cuff muscles. There are some patients who have a true mechanical reason for their pain—a narrower outlet for the tendon or arthritis in the overlying joint that swells, causing spurs or otherwise constricting the space available for the rotator cuff. But these cases are less common than the patient with shoulder pain and a perfectly normal x-ray. Surgery is less likely to help the patient who has nothing really structurally wrong with the shoulder.

Complete Rotator Cuff Tears

Complete tears of the rotator cuff tendon are actually rare in this age group. They certainly can occur and, when they do, surgical repair is the only real treatment. But more often than not when people arrive in my office, the cuff is just in the early stages of wearing out and responds nicely to non-operative modalities.

The real gray zone and the controversial issue is what to do about what we call "partial thickness cuff tears." Most surgeons agree that any midlife patient who has a complete cuff tear should have it fixed surgically. We may come to blows over whether this is best done with the tried- and-

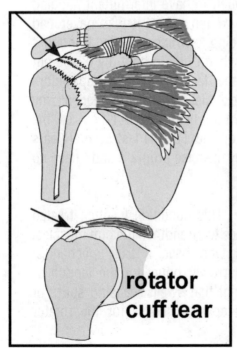

rotator cuff tear

true open procedure or through the newer arthroscopic techniques, but one way or another we would all fix a completely torn cuff. But what about these partial thickness tears that you only know about because they show up on MRI? Should they be fixed? Can they be fixed? Should you wait until they tear completely and then fix them? Should you go in arthroscopically and "debride" them, (which means, literally, "to cut away"—French jargon, in this case), or should you open up the shoulder and repair them directly? These are all unanswered questions. Most of us are conservative enough to treat most partial thickness cuff tears with exercises and activity modification as opposed to surgery, but there are many articulate arguments for at least arthroscopic debridement in those that have failed to respond to a legitimate trial of non-operative management.

This is one place where the surgical techniques are evolving. There is a trend away from open repairs of true rotator cuff tears and toward more arthroscopic, or "less invasive," techniques. But buyer, beware! Some surgeons will scope your shoulder first and then open it anyway to do the repair. I personally don't think the shoulder should be scoped just because it's there, when there is scant indication for operative intervention. I may be out on limb here with my colleagues, but I recommend a persistent conservative management of these problems before considering surgery. There is no question that there are good indications for arthroscopic shoulder surgery. I'm just saying that the indication is not simply a case of "painful shoulder".

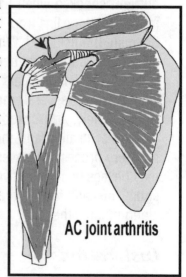

AC joint arthritis

As I mentioned earlier, there are specific anatomic conditions that contribute to rotator cuff tendonitis and pain, such as arthritis in the joint between the collarbone and shoulder blade, a joint that lies right above the cuff.

Spurs from this "acromioclavicular" (or AC) joint may

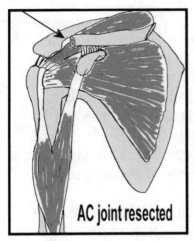

AC joint resected

rub on the tendon. When conservative treatment for this condition is unsuccessful, surgery to remove the spurs is warranted. This too can be done either with traditional open surgery or with arthroscopic techniques. Here again, it's critical to know the training and experience of your surgeon.

One of the hardest things for boomers to swallow is that all these shoulder conditions take a long time to get over, whether treated with or without surgery. The recovery from surgery for a complete rotator cuff tear, for instance, will take around six months and at times up to a year. So the boomer looking for a quick fix is going to be disappointed if not outright shocked when I tell him what he's getting into. I'm reminded of the line from Monty Python, "No one expects the Spanish Inquisition!" Who among us is ready to go six weeks after surgery without actively lifting the arm (while the rotator cuff tendon heals back down), and then follow that with another several months of gradual strengthening? Unfortunately, arthroscopic repair doesn't really change the biology of healing and therefore doesn't really shorten this recovery process. It leaves a smaller scar or scars and there may be less post-operative pain in the early period, but in the end, "You can't fool Mother Nature." And you can't hustle her along much either.

Dislocations

One price the shoulder pays for its remarkable mobility is its tendency to come out of place—to dislocate. Here another definition or two will be helpful. When a joint goes completely out of place (in this case the ball coming completely out of the socket), we call that a *dislocation*. When a joint slides or goes just partially out of place, we call that a *subluxation*. Both these conditions occur with some frequency around the shoulder. I will describe dislocations of the shoulder joint proper (the glenohumeral joint) and then dislocations of the joint where the collarbone meets the shoulder blade (the acromioclavicular joint). These latter dislocations are sometimes called shoulder "separations". Both are common and commonly confused with each other.

Glenohumeral (Shoulder) Dislocations

I see many boomers who started having shoulder dislocations in their youth, usually the mid-teenage years at fifteen, sixteen, or seventeen years of age. They were footballers, wrestlers, swimmers etc., in a word, jocks or risk-takers. Usually there was originally one legitimate traumatic event that got this all started. Let's say Steve was a linebacker and dislocated his shoulder first when he was a junior in high school. The first time it was incredibly painful and he had to be carried off the field and taken to the emergency room where the doctor sedated him and put it back in. Then it was fine, though every now and then it would come out again. But eventually it was easier to get back in. The trainer could do it for him. A few times, he'd dislocate during the big game and Marty the trainer would pull on it for him, pop it back in and he'd not only play the rest of the game, he'd go to the

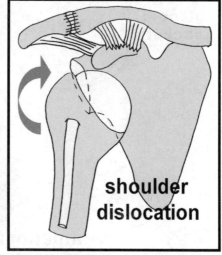

shoulder dislocation

dance afterwards.

Then it calmed down and, while he was focusing on his studies in college, he noticed it never went completely out. But sometimes, particularly when he tried to put his arm up over his head, like getting into a T-shirt or sometimes while sleeping, it would *almost* go out. Lately, it's been getting more painful and less predictable. He's learned to avoid certain positions, but he's bothered by the fact that he can't play ball with his kids, and he's worried that someday he'll be in Belize sleeping in a hammock and wake up with a dislocated shoulder that the local shaman might not be able to get it back in.

What's going on here is that the original injury that dislocated his shoulder tore the restraining ligaments away from the front of the socket. These ligaments are strong bands of tissue that start on the front of the socket and cross over the front of the ball to anchor into the head of the humerus.

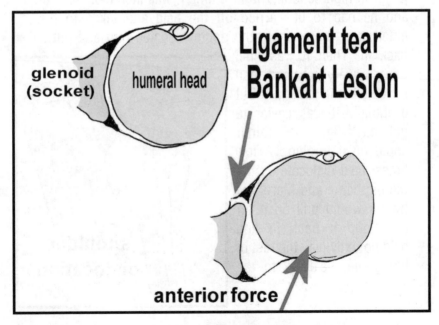

The first dislocation back in high school tore those ligaments away from their anchorage on the socket. So now whenever the arm goes up and out, they can't restrain the shoulder—the ligaments are all lax and stretched out—and the ball starts to slide out of the socket in front. It may only subluxate or it may frankly dislocate, but neither feels good and either is a good reason to get it fixed.

The surgical correction for this condition is a repair of the ligaments in the front of the shoulder, re-establishing their attachment on the front rim of the socket and sometimes strengthening the stretched out ligaments by overlapping them or even using radio-frequency tissue cooking techniques to shrink them. This is another area where the exact surgical techniques are currently evolving, and that always means there will be two camps of surgeons. On the conservative side will be mostly balding and gray-haired doctors recommending open repair through tried and true techniques that have stood the test of time. *And in this corner!* Mostly eager, bright-eyed young guys with a few months or perhaps years of experience with the latest, so-called minimally invasive technique.

Though I'm sure my bias stands out like sour cream on a tuxedo sleeve, I have to admit all the advances ever made in surgery have been made by those eager

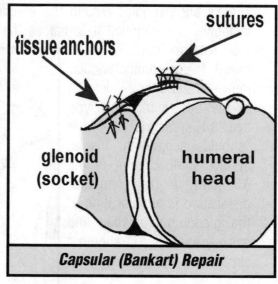

sutures

tissue anchors

glenoid (socket)

humeral head

Capsular (Bankart) Repair

beavers with a new technique—but so have most of the biggest disasters. As a patient you just have to decide whether you want to be one of those pioneering souls who buys into what is yet to be proven to work over time. Informed consent is the name of the game. Whatever you choose, you should want to know how long this technique has been around, how many have been done, how long the follow-up is and how the results compare to standard, usually open, techniques. And those are the same questions we should be asking ourselves as surgeons before we strike off into uncharted territory.

There's a great joke among surgeons about what we call "Christopher Columbus Surgery." "Hell," said the wise old surgeon, "that looks like a Christopher Columbus case to me. He didn't know where he was going when he started; he didn't know where he was when he got there; and he didn't know where he'd been when he got back."

Shoulder Separations

There's another joint around the shoulder that's prone to instability. I mentioned it earlier as the roof that lies over the rotator cuff. This is called the acromioclavicular joint—affectionately known as the "AC" joint. When you hear of someone having a "shoulder separation," that is, in fact, a dislocation of the AC joint. A true shoulder dislocation is a dislocation of the glenohumeral (ball and socket) joint, and a shoulder separation is a dislocation

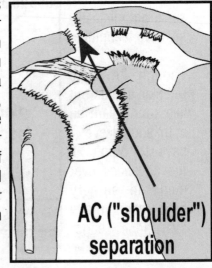

AC ("shoulder") separation

of that joint where the clavicle (collarbone) meets the acromion (part of the shoulder blade).

Just as shoulder function is an interplay of those three muscle groups I talked about earlier, the bony anatomy involves three genuine joints and one very important imposter.

Of the three genuine joints you've already met two: the glenohumeral joint (the ball and socket) and the AC joint. The third is actually the only place where the whole upper extremity is attached to the rest of the axial (central) skeleton. This is at the medial end of the clavicle, where it attaches to the sternum (breastbone) at what is called the sternoclavicular (SC) joint. So you have the clavicle attached to the sternum at one end, the shoulder blade suspended from the clavicle by the AC joint at the other end, and the shoulder blade attached to the arm by the glenohumeral joint. "The arm bone's connected to the shoulder bone; the shoulder bone's connected to the collarbone; the collarbone's connected to the breast bone." At each joint there are strong ligaments that keep the joint in place and support this whole relationship, the purpose of which, as you remember, is mobility. The goal is to place the hand anywhere the owner wants to place it (hopefully within reason and within some social constraints). Luckily there are few afflictions of the sternoclavicular joint and almost none of those affect Boomers, so I can move on to that fourth, unconventional joint.

The fourth joint that controls shoulder motion is not really a joint in the true sense of the word, but it is responsible for almost half the combined motion of the shoulder. Unlike true joints that (1) have bone ends that meet together restrained by formal ligaments, (2) are covered with joint cartilage and

85

(3) are bathed in joint fluid, this fourth joint is held together only by muscles. It has no ligaments, joint cartilage or joint fluid. This pseudo-joint occurs where the shoulder blade meets and moves against the chest wall or thorax and is called the "scapulothoracic joint." Here the scapula moves and rotates while held against the upper chest wall by the strong muscles I previously described as the basses or scapular stabilizers. This relatively free motion of the scapula against the chest is responsible for almost half of what we think of as shoulder motion. The glenohumeral joint is responsible for the other half. A person can completely lose all motion in the glenohumeral joint—as happens in the case of a "frozen shoulder"—but he will still have about half of his shoulder motion left, the half that comes from the motion of the scapula against the chest. We'll come back to the critical importance of this scapulothoracic joint later when we discuss frozen shoulder.

In shoulder separations, the mechanism of injury that sprains the AC joint is a fall on the tip of the shoulder. Football, soccer and rugby, sports in which players tumble and wind up ass-over-tea-kettle, are all especially good at causing this injury. Thus, boomers in the fitness-as-competition and risk-taker syndrome groups are especially prone to this problem. But this also happens with great frequency in such activities as cycling and roller-blading. I've even seen one klutz sustain this injury when he fell off a moving treadmill.

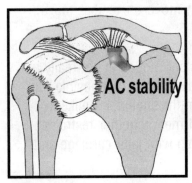
AC stability

Whatever the mechanism, an AC joint sprain depresses the shoulder blade away from its articulation with the collarbone by forcibly separating the two, leaving the arm hanging freely, unsuspended at its usual tether from the clavicle. This may look like the collarbone is sticking up toward the ear, but, in fact, the collar bones are still at the same horizontal level. What's going on is that the weight of the arm is pulling down on the whole complex. The arm and the shoulder blade are still attached

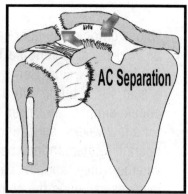

at the glenohumeral joint, but the whole business has become dissociated from the clavicle at the sprained AC joint and is dragged down by the weight of the arm.

The treatment for this varies. Though this may seem like an obviously out-of-whack situation—and if ever something looked as if it needed to be fixed, this is it—in truth, these injuries do very well left without surgical treatment. Even the more severe cases rarely wind up with much pain. In general, we put these into a sling and, when the pain starts to die down, we start moving the shoulder. Even most professional athletes are treated without surgery. However, there are some patients who should be operated on to repair the torn ligaments and restore stability to this joint. These are mostly heavy laborers or people who do a lot of lifting. We don't fix most athletes because they are so muscular that the deformity from this is barely noticeable and the loss of strength is negligible . . . and they'll just tear it up again anyway. I can think of several NBA players

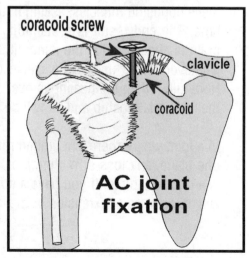

whose chronic shoulder separations show up larger than life on your big screen home TV, especially when they step up to the free-throw line. Some skinny people who prefer to trade a scar for a bump should probably be fixed, but most people simply don't need it. I generally follow people along for a few weeks, educating them about the pros and cons of operative intervention, before letting them help me decide whether they should have an operation. The operation involves screwing the collarbone back down to the shoulder blade and reconstructing the ligaments that are ruptured. And like all shoulder operations it involves a recovery of several months.

The Frozen Shoulder

The body treats pain in almost any joint in the same way. It immobilizes it with a combination of muscle spasm and swelling in the joint and the adjacent tissues. The message from the brain is: "Stop moving this or I'll hurt you." Muscle groups that act in opposite ways across the same joint are normally wired so that when one contracts, the other relaxes. Tighten the muscle that extends the knee and you're supposed to relax the one that flexes it and so forth. When the joint in question is injured, the brain fires off impulses to these opposing muscles, asking both to contract at the same time. The end result is a standoff, and that's just what the brain is after. It holds the joint still, so it can begin to repair whatever is the underlying cause of that painful stimulus. Hopefully, when the healing is over, the muscles can resume their old relationship and all will be well.

In a joint where there is a limited range of motion, usually in one plane, any loss of motion is noticeable. Again, the knee is a good example. If you have a sore knee and you lose the last 15 degrees of extension or the last 30 degrees of flexion, you notice it right away. It's a stiff knee and you know there's something wrong that needs attention, and soon. It's the same with the elbow or the finger joints or almost any other joint you can name. But the shoulder has so much motion that you can lose a large part of it and almost not notice. Remember that half of the combined motion of the shoulder comes from the scapulothoracic joint, so you can have lost all of the glenohumeral (ball and socket) joint motion and still retain a lot of shoulder motion. This is exactly what happens in the condition we call frozen shoulder.

Frozen shoulder is one of those diagnoses that in a way is not a diagnosis at all. It's a description of the final common pathway of anything that causes shoulder pain to the point that the patient has stopped moving it and it has gotten stiff. You can get a frozen shoulder from a rotator cuff tendonitis, from a fracture almost anywhere in the upper extremity, from a hand injury, from being in a cast for some other injury in the upper extremity, from breast surgery, from a pinched nerve in the neck and from a host of other things. Whatever the original painful stimulus, the common denominator is a glenohumeral joint that hasn't moved through its normally expansive range or motion and usually for quite some time. Often by the time the patient sees me with a stiff shoulder, the original cause is lost to antiquity.

I saw a woman only a little older than I am who had been referred to me by a general surgeon. He was concerned that one of her shoulder nerves might have been injured during a reconstructive breast procedure, done after mastectomy for cancer. This type of surgery often involves dissection and removal of the lymph nodes in the armpit. In this case, that was the original painful stimulus. I was seeing her months after the fact and, although the breast reconstruction had worked out quite well cosmetically, the patient couldn't lift her arm. Both her plastic surgeon and her cancer surgeon were concerned.

After I took her history, I was pretty sure what I'd find when I examined her. I asked her to raise her hand up in front as high as she could, then out to the side as far as she could, then to reach behind her back as far as she could and so on. In all respects she demonstrated about half of normal active shoulder motion. When I held her shoulder blade still against her chest wall by pushing down from above (thereby eliminating motion from the scapulothoracic joint), then tried to move her arm at the glenohumeral joint, there was almost no motion. The shoulder was "frozen" at the glenohumeral joint. This was not a nerve problem; this was a classic frozen shoulder. And believe me, all involved were glad that it was the latter.

The ten-dollar doctors' term for frozen shoulder is "adhesive capsulitis," but in many ways the layman's term is more appropriate. Adhesive capsulitis implies that the shoulder joint capsule or those ligaments that hold the ball near the socket have become inflamed and that somehow that is the underlying mechanism of the loss of motion. Well, maybe that happens sometimes, but most of the time there is little or no inflammation at all. It's just a contracted joint that has arisen as the ligaments have shortened through lack of motion. The same thing happens to the knee if we put it in a cast for six weeks, but we don't call that "adhesive capsulitis" of the knee.

No matter what you call it, you still have to thaw it. The treatment for frozen shoulder is gradual stretching and mobilization. At first this may be best done under supervision of a therapist, but as quickly as possible the patient has to come to understand that he or she is the real therapist. Only the patient can stretch out that shoulder. Some orthopedists feel strongly about never sending these patients to the therapist, but in these cases I think we are acting on the old adage that "all politics are local." Whether or not your doctor recommends you to a physical therapist really depends on the quality of the therapists in your local environment—and partly on the patient. Many would do better with just a few therapy sessions, some with none at all. I find that most of my boomer patients do best when I start them out with a physical therapist and then allow them to transition to doing the stretches on their own.

There is little room for surgery in the treatment of frozen shoulder; but, once again, there are specific indications for surgically manipulating the shoulder or, in some cases, performing open or arthroscopic resection of the adhesions inside the joint. I manipulate about one out of every twenty frozen shoulders that I see, and most of those are diabetics. For various reasons, diabetes is a stiffening disease, so we commonly see frozen shoulders in diabetic patients. If a patient has made little or no progress with a good trial of physical therapy, I think putting them to sleep and carefully putting the shoulder through a controlled stretch to break up the joint adhesions is a legitimate thing to do. This carries the risk of breaking something other than just the adhesions and I tell patients that my biggest concern with this manipulation is that I'll hear a crack just before the motion improves dramatically. But I add that, so far, I've never fractured a humerus by manipulating the shoulder.

Through the years, I've treated many physicians for this condition. One was a surgeon who limbered up one shoulder, only to have "the same damn thing" start up in the other shoulder. This is not uncommon. A frozen shoulder can take six months to a year to thaw and the chance of it occurring on both sides is at least twenty percent. Surprisingly, the most common symptom is not really the loss of motion, but pain at night. I think this is because when you toss and turn at night, the stiff shoulder is forced to the end of its range of movement and the pain wakes the patient up. Luckily, that pain during the night is also usually one of the first things to get better with the standard treatment of stretching and the "tincture of time."

Fractures Around the Shoulder

There can be any number of fracture combinations involving the three bones that participate in the joints around the shoulder. I'll focus on the most common fractures that we see in the boomer population: fractures of the clavicle and fractures of the upper end of the arm bone (the proximal humerus). Fractures of the scapula are rare and, with the exception of those that involve the socket part, usually quite benign.

Most of the injuries to the shoulder that result in fractures involve falls. Falls from bicycles, falls from a height, falls while skiing, falls while roller-blading, falls down the stairs—there are just a thousand ways to demonstrate the Law of

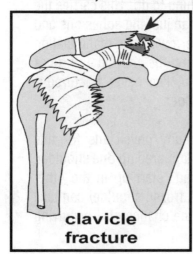

Gravity. Falls from bicycles are particularly common, especially with the increase in cycling sports, triathalons, cycle touring vacations etc.

When I was in private practice in Burlington, Iowa in the 1980s, the famous RAGBRAI (*The Des Moines Register's Annual Great Bike Ride Across Iowa*) would

clavicle fracture

sometimes end up in Burlington. This wonderful bacchanal always begins on one side of the state at the Missouri River and rolls for a week across the Iowa summer prairie, ending seven days later at some town on the Mississippi River. Along the way, riders would stop at every little farm town and hamlet, have some sweet corn or some fresh rhubarb pie and usually a beer or two—just to wash it down. Then they'd camp out each night, have barbecue and, well, maybe a few more beers—just to wash it down. By week's end this crowd of cyclists would number in the thousands and the number of headaches and hangovers would be substantial as well. Just before you enter Burlington on the main highway from the north there is a huge downhill. It's the kind of hill that sneaks up on you. It starts out gradually and then builds up more and more momentum until you find yourself racing along *with the wind in you hair!* And what have we learned about feeling the wind in your hair? You've guessed it exactly: there is a *Life Altering Event* right around the corner, sure as shootin'. My second year there, RAGBRAI came over that hill and piled up a whole bunch of riders, and I was in the ER treating fractured clavicles.

Luckily, the treatment for a fractured clavicle is usually a sling at first, and then a figure-of-eight strap that goes around both shoulders and pulls them into a sort of military position with the shoulders back. After a few weeks, the pain subsides and the break usually knits with a slight bump in the middle of the collarbone that just never quite goes away. Children heal this fracture in a few weeks. But in about ten or fifteen percent of adults, the thing will either not heal or begins to heal in such a crooked position that I'll have to go in and put a plate and screws across it, leaving an unavoidable scar along most of the length of the bone. Suffice it to say, this injury is best treated by simple prevention.

By prevention I mean the following: 1) if you're cycling, avoid your neighbors or allow enough separation around you so that you don't have to pay for someone else's screw-up. 2) Never go up on a ladder without a spotter. This includes the standard six-foot stepladder. I can't tell you how many people I've seen ride one of these babies down and come up with a broken something. 3) If you ski, ski within your limits and never take that last run on the last day of the vacation. Just go in and sit by the fire and tell stories. 4) Finally, don't go up or down a flight of stairs in the dark, especially if you wear bifocals. Eventually you'll miss a step and nothing good will come of it.

Now these may seem like silly admonitions for an otherwise young, healthy boomer population, but I can give you multiple examples of how each of the above resulted in what I would consider an avoidable, painful, and sometimes surgical fracture of the clavicle.

All of the same advice could apply to prevention of the next fracture group, those that involve the upper end of the arm bone or humerus. In the lingo we call these "fractures of the proximal humerus."

These are often sustained in higher velocity injuries such as motor vehicle accidents and falls from even greater heights.

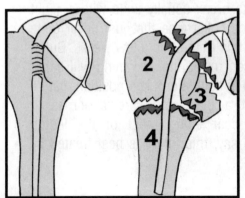

Recently, I've seen a few of these from jet ski accidents. In Minnesota and Iowa it was the snowmobile and in California it's those dirt bikes and all-terrain vehicles that they race around in the desert, tearing up the turf. The Modern American Male has shown endless inventiveness in marrying the internal combustion engine to vehicular mayhem. To me these are all variations on a theme. The first time I heard a jet ski coming around the bend I thought, "Damn, that sounds like a snowmobile out on the water." And in a way, that's just what it is.

The proximal humerus fractures when it is forced against the socket violently or when all the muscles contract at once and hold the ball rigidly in the socket as the rest of the arm tries to keep moving. These fractures are often badly displaced in our age group and frequently require big operations to fix and hold the parts in place. Sometimes fractures here are combined with dislocations. The good news is that with all its inherent motion, the shoulder is one joint that can take a joke. It can heal with some displacement and some stiffness and still function pretty well. But it may not allow the patient to return to full sporting activities. The bad news is that almost all fractures that can't be treated in a simple sling require open operations, significant scars and usually have a prolonged recovery period.

So once again, it might be best to assess your high-risk physical behaviors. A little less Evil Knievel and little more Thoreau might be the way to go.

Chapter 5: The Elbow

This is a story about the elbow that starts with a story about brain surgery. Hang in there. Remember the Brain[5] always has to have its say.

One of my colleagues in the Air Force was a spine surgeon named Jim. He seemed to have more than his share of medical problems, including an injury he sustained boxing while a student at the Air Force Academy. He fractured the small bone at the base of the skull where the olfactory nerves pass from the brain to the nose. These are the nerves that transmit the sense of smell. Fracturing this bone is like pulling a plug in the bottom of the sink that is the brain, letting the spinal fluid slowly leak into the nose. This happened so slowly and subtly in his case that he thought the stuff coming out his nose was due to allergies. After college and medical school he was in the middle of his internship when he started getting high fevers and terrible headaches. In other words, only after he had developed meningitis (a brain infection!) did he realize what was going on. This required an operation where the neurosurgeons went in and lifted up his brain to patch the leaky floor underneath. Unfortunately, this operation plucked out those olfactory nerves leaving my friend the spine surgeon unable to smell anything for the rest of his life.

What does all this have to do with the elbow? Well, I'll explain. While we were together at Wilford Hall Medical Center in San Antonio, Jim developed tennis elbow from the peculiar position in which spine surgeons have to use certain instruments and the unique stresses this places on the elbow. We injected it, cast it, did all the right things, but it wouldn't go away. He eventually had to have surgery to repair

---

5 I've capitalized "Brain" in this narrative and other places throughout the book where it becomes a character rather than just another organ.

it. He was in his post-operative cast when the opportunity of a lifetime came knocking. Jim was a career officer and as a career officer in the medical corps the ultimate validation is to be a war surgeon. In 1989 we were both staff orthopedists at Wilford Hall when the USA decided to teach Manuel Noriega and those pesky Panamanians a lesson. The lesson was called "Operation Just Cause." One morning at 0400 we got the call that we'd invaded Panama and the casualties were on their way to us. In the next few hours we admitted over a hundred soldiers with fresh-off-the-battlefield injuries. Over 90% had orthopedic injuries: parachute mishaps, high-velocity gunshot wounds, fractures and shrapnel. We operated our butts off for the next week and there was

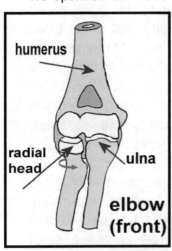

humerus

radial head

ulna

elbow (front)

Jim in his cast, missing the dance. He later told me that the damn tennis elbow caused him much more grief than his meningitis, the brain surgery, or even not being able to smell ever did.

Like the shoulder, the elbow is a common source of pain among boomers. Although tennis elbow is by far the most common problem, a few other aggravations arise in this spot halfway between the shoulder and the hand. I'll begin by reviewing the pertinent anatomy and go from there to the specific problems that I treat.

The Anatomy of the Elbow

The elbow results from the articulation of three bones: the humerus or arm bone above, and the two forearm bones, the radius and the ulna, below. In fact, the primary function of the elbow is to act as the hinge joint between the humerus and the ulna. This hinge has motion in only one plane. The elbow straightens as the ulna swings down from the humerus and it bends up as the ulna swings up toward the humerus. We call the

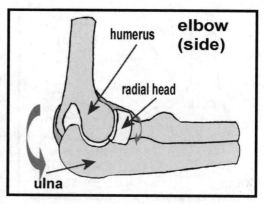

straightening "extension" and the bending upward "flexion." Thus, we speak of the elbow as extending and flexing at the joint between the humerus and the ulna.

There is a second part of the elbow where the radius rotates inside the elbow joint and against the humerus, allowing the forearm to rotate as the mobile radius rotates around the stationary ulna. This arrangement allows the elbow to assist the shoulder in multiplying the wonderful complexity of positions that the human hand can reach. We'll see later how the wrist and hand multiply this effect even more. But the variety of positions allowed through combined shoulder and elbow motion allow even a stiff wrist or hand to remain remarkably functional. It is no surprise that the versatile mechanical manipulator on the Space Shuttle is called the "Robot Arm" and not the "Robot Leg." It is, in fact, designed on many of the same principles as the human upper extremity. You could call this a case of God making Man, who then made Robot in His own image.

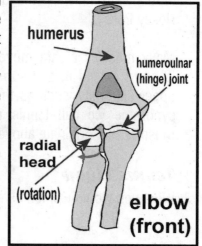

Each of the two parts of the elbow

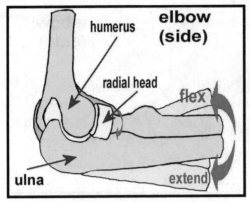

joint is designed to suit its unique purpose. The humero-ulnar joint is a constrained hinge with a concave scoop on the upper end of the ulna that fits perfectly into the convex spool on the end of the humerus.

Sitting right next to this, and still within the elbow joint capsule, is the humero-radial joint, designed for rotation. The upper end of the radius is a circular plate that rotates against a corresponding ball on the end of the humerus. This allows for rotation of the radius in almost any degree of flexion or extension. You can prove this to yourself by straightening out your elbow and turning your hand over palm up and then palm down. Now flex your elbow completely and do the same thing. Remarkable, huh? You also get an idea what a room full of medical students taking an anatomy exam looks like. Imagine a lecture hall full of highly educated, self-directed gunners, twisting and turning in their seats, trying to feel this or that tendon or bony prominence and doing what I call the "Anatomy Hokey Pokey."

Many muscles create movement of the elbow. Some flex it, some extend it, and some have duties farther down the upper extremity, such as those that move the wrist. In the syndrome we call tennis elbow, it's these wrist-moving muscles that originate above the elbow that get in trouble.

Tennis Elbow

What you would call tennis elbow, I call lateral epicondylitis.

The lateral epicondyle is that bump on the outside of your elbow that is the anchor for the origin of the muscles that extend your wrist and fingers.

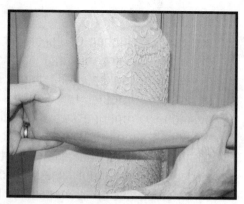

Inflammation of that muscle origin is called epicondylitis, and it most commonly occurs on the outer side of the elbow, hence the term lateral epicondylitis. This condition is so common it is almost universal. I suspect less than half the patients who experience this ever get bad enough to see their doctor, and an even smaller percentage of those ever get to some specialist like me. When they do, they typically complain of pain over the outside of the elbow that worsens with lifting, gives them difficulty turning doorknobs and carrying their briefcase or luggage, causes problems at the computer, and sometimes pain with just writing. By the time they come to see me, their symptoms have usually been going on for months and they may have tried all or some of the usual treatments: anti-inflammatory medicines, a forearm band (tennis-elbow strap), and maybe even an injection or two of cortisone.

In spite of the name, this classic overuse or strain syndrome almost never comes from tennis. In fact, it's usually only amateur tennis players with a poor backhand technique who get this. Pros get the same thing but on the other side, the flexor side of their elbow, and then it's from their powerful forehand. Most of us duffers get tennis elbow from doing something over and over for which the human machine was just not designed. If you look back at our history, we evolved through learning how to survive by our wits. We crouched at the edge of the savannah, waited for the wildebeest to wander by, clubbed or speared him, dragged him a short distance, cut him up, dragged the remains back to camp, made a fire, cooked a little dinner, and so on. We sure didn't sit at the computer for eight or ten hours a day in one position, hammering away. We didn't sit scrunched into a dollhouse airline seat with a laptop perched on our knees, plunking out a business report. God apparently didn't envision the assembly line with one woman screwing one screw clockwise on every passing DVD player, once every 20 seconds for four hours at a time.

The underlying pathology of tennis elbow is a disruption of the bony anchor of the origin of that group of muscles that pull up the wrist and hand. As I sit here typing this paragraph on my computer, I am in exactly the position that both provokes this and makes it so persistent. Most everything we do is with the hand extended at the wrist. So once this syndrome gets started, it is typically chronic and uniquely aggravating. I tell my frustrated patients that although no one ever dies from this, many wish they had.

The good news is that epicondylitis almost always goes away over time, no matter what we do. The bad news is that it can last up to a year, and that can be one miserable year. The standard treatments are the usual anti-inflammatories, a strap that you wear around the forearm to redistribute the hydraulic muscle forces away from the muscle origin, cortisone shots to further relieve the inflammation and stretching exercises to reduce the strain on the muscle anchor. In cases that fail to improve after the first cortisone injection, I'll often combine a second injection with a brief period in a cast, putting the musculotendinous unit to rest. This procedure is often effective where injection alone is not. Surgery is reserved for those patients who have failed conservative management for several months. For every 50 people with this condition that we see, we operate on one or two. When necessary, the surgery involves releasing the muscle origin from the scar tissue that has formed underneath it and, in general, repairing the damage. This procedure usually involves several weeks of immobilization after surgery. This is the stage where my friend Jim was when George Bush decided to exercise the Monroe Doctrine.

Ulnar Neuropathy at the Elbow

The most famous nerve in the upper extremity is the one that gets pinched at the wrist in carpal tunnel syndrome, the median nerve. We'll talk about that nerve later, but you have probably already experienced first hand

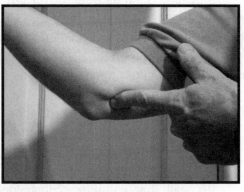

its close cousin, the completely misnamed "funny bone," or ulnar nerve. When you whack your so-called funny bone, you're actually contusing the ulnar nerve where it passes behind the medial side of the elbow. If you feel there, you'll find a little ditch between the humerus and ulna bones.

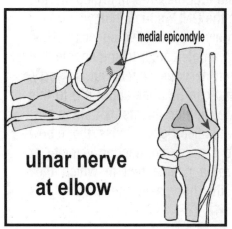

medial epicondyle

ulnar nerve at elbow

This is perhaps best felt with the elbow at half-mast. In this ditch lies the nerve that goes to the small and ring fingers and most of the small muscles of the hand. When you suddenly bump the ulnar nerve in this groove, it shoots an excruciating pain down the ulnar side of the forearm and into the hand. The nerve is actually pretty well protected in its little trough, so it takes a real dumb move to smash it, but when you do, there's nothing funny about it.

This arrangement may protect the ulnar nerve from most insults, but because it has to pass over such a bony prominence as the elbow, in some people it becomes sensitive or irritated. This may have to do with direct pressure, such as truck drivers or other vehicular operators experience when they have to rest their forearms and elbows on their arm rests. Constant pressure on the medial side of the elbow will eventually show up as symptoms downstream where the ulnar nerve goes. The symptom at first is mainly numbness in the areas that the ulnar nerve supplies: the small and ring fingers. Irritation of this nerve eventually progresses, resulting in symptoms of weakness in the small muscles of the hand that are responsible for pinch and grip.

We call this condition "ulnar neuropathy" or alternately, "ulnar nerve entrapment." The first trick in treating it is recognizing it and distinguishing it from the other things that can cause numbness in this distribution, namely a pinched nerve in the neck or a pinching of the ulnar nerve farther along at the wrist. Here, our buddies the neurologists are helpful. (In fact, this may be the ONLY situation in which they are helpful, theirs being largely a descriptive specialty. How would you like to spend your whole career telling people that this or that is wrong with their nervous system but, so sorry, there really isn't anything that can be done about it?) In this situation, at least they can do the nerve tests that show how the ulnar nerve conducts its electricity across the elbow and the wrist. This is called a nerve conduction velocity or NCV. They can also perform a needle test in which they evaluate the way each of the nerves in the extremity is conducting its electricity to a given muscle. This is called an electromyogram or EMG. By combining EMGs and NCVs they can tell us whether this problem is, in fact, really an ulnar neuropathy at the elbow or the wrist or, simply a pinched nerve in the neck, masquerading as such.

Patients are often very impressed with these "electro-diagnostic" tests. Some come back to my office thinking they've had some kind of magical treatment. Through the years, I've had a number of patients tell me about "those shock treatments" that I sent them for and how they cured the problem. They probably say this because nobody would want to have this test done twice. In any event, these tests are often critical in making the diagnosis in this and most other nerve compression problems in the upper extremity.

Once the diagnosis is established, and as long as there is no weakness, only numbness, the initial treatment involves educating the patient to avoid pressure on that side of the elbow. Often this includes nighttime splinting to keep the elbow from flexing completely. This position of full flexion places the ulnar nerve under maximum stretch and may set off the problem. Patients can either be fitted with a splint made in the orthopedist's cast room or a custom brace made at the brace shop. They can even use the simpler technique of wrapping a towel around their elbow inside of an ace wrap. This little bolster somehow reminds the sleeping elbow not to flex all the way. My wife, Kathy, actually had bilateral ulnar neuropathy for a while. Every time she went to sleep her small and ring fingers would go numb. We fitted her with little foam elbow pads that she put on when she slept. They limited her elbow flexion just enough to relieve the condition.

For those patients who present with frank weakness in the muscles supplied by the ulnar nerve, or who fail treatment with splinting and avoidance of pressure, surgery may be necessary. This surgery involves moving the nerve from behind the elbow to in front of it. Called an "ulnar nerve transposition," this works by shortening the distance the nerve has to travel, lessening the effects of prolonged flexion and getting it out of that position behind the elbow where it is vulnerable to pressure when we rest our forearm on a surface. This is like putting the ulnar nerve on a direct flight rather than having it make a connection in Atlanta. Ulnar nerve transposition is an outpatient procedure that involves a significant scar (about six inches long) but the results are usually gratifying. Most people get better over time, but not quickly like patients with a carpal tunnel release. Many take several months to recover, and some who have dense numbness before surgery will only get minimal improvement. But, hopefully, they will be able to avoid the inevitable weakness that can occur if this condition is left untreated.

Olecranon Bursitis

Since this is not the first time we've come across the term "bursitis," I suppose it's high time I explained the anatomy of a bursa. "Bursa" comes from the Latin word for wine skin. In the body, the bursae function as lubricators and friction

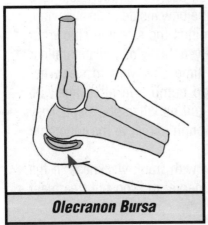

Olecranon Bursa

handlers. Anywhere that two surfaces come into friction or opposition, or where there is movement between two crossing muscles, such as a muscle across a bone, you will find a bursa. They handle friction. I think of them as the marriage counselors of the body. *Dorland's Medical*

Dictionary lists two and half pages of bursae—-roughly equivalent to the New Orleans Yellow Pages list of family counselors. The two most famous are the one in the shoulder that used to get incriminated as a cause of shoulder pain, and the one that lies over the prominence of the elbow. This latter is called the "olecranon bursa" because it provides a lubricated sack that lets the skin of the elbow move freely over the prominence of the ulna bone, which we call the olecranon.

All bursae are more or less little sacks of the same sort of tissue that lines the joints. Just like joints, they can produce a lubricating synovial fluid that allows near frictionless motion of our moving parts. I tell my patients to think of a bursa as a small, collapsed balloon with just a few drops of fluid inside. In this state bursae facilitate motion while taking up very little space. They can lie between almost any two surfaces that experience friction. The problem arises when something irritates the bursa. Being specialized, a bursa is a one-trick pony. Surgeons are accused of the same crime, by the way. "To a man with a hammer, everything looks like a nail[6]," is the joke about the surgeon who sees *only* a surgical solution for any problem. The bursa has a repertoire of exactly one response: it can make more fluid. Bump it too hard—it makes more fluid. Rub it too long and too much—it makes more fluid. In a tight space like the shoulder, this extra fluid may limit motion and cause pain. Under the flabby skin over the elbow, it just makes an unsightly bump that can grow to the size of an egg.

At first, this egg is painless and is little more than an ugly sack hanging off the back of the elbow. Over time, if it isn't treated, it may either get infected or the bursa wall will thicken to the point where it is no longer just a fluid filled balloon, but more like a hard-boiled egg of fibrous tissue.

6   This is usually attributed to Mark Twain.

Both of these situations require surgical removal. You often see these thickened, chronic olecranon bursae on the elbows of alcoholics, presumably from resting their arms on the bar for years. For this reason, this condition is sometimes called "beer drinker's elbow," not a pretty appellation.

At the initial presentation of symptoms, olecranon bursitis can be treated with aspiration (sticking a needle into it to drain the extra fluid) and compression. I believe compression is the key. If the doctor simply drains the bursa, but doesn't put a wrap or elastic sleeve around it to prevent it from re-accumulating fluid, the problem is almost guaranteed to come right back. Sometimes I'll combine an aspiration with immobilization by putting the elbow to rest in a cast for a week. This almost always guarantees the resolution of the problem.

There is some risk in leaving this condition untreated. The synovial fluid in an olecranon bursa is a great medium for growing bacteria. Left untreated, these commonly get infected and, once infected, more commonly require surgery and excision. But these rank more as aggravations than surgical urgencies.

Fractures

Broken elbows are bad news. Luckily, the most common breaks are those around the radial head, the rotating upper end of the radius. These come in several flavors, and the minor ones are more common than the major ones, but almost any fracture around the elbow can result in loss of motion. The elbow is a very constrained joint. The more constrained or tighter the tolerances in a joint, the less it can take a joke. As you remember, the shoulder is a sloppy, mobile joint with motion all over the place, and it tolerates injury surprisingly well. The elbow is the exact opposite. It is so tightly fit, that almost any displacement of the fractured parts will result in a loss of function. Even an undisplaced fracture (a hairline crack) can result in a loss of motion.

All fractures within a joint cause bleeding into that joint. Since the joint is a self-contained sack of synovium, this extra fluid causes both a painful distention and a loss

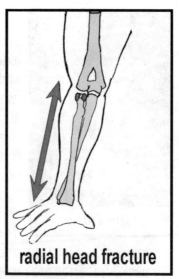

radial head fracture

of motion. Let's take the boomer who falls from his bicycle and breaks the fall with his outstretched hand. The elbow is usually locked in its fully extended position and the force of the fall is transmitted up the wrist through the radius and to the radial head, which is forced against the humerus, fracturing the radial head.

This may be a way-out-of-whack displaced fracture that causes a mechanical block to elbow motion and needs surgery. Or it may be just a hairline crack that causes no mechanical block to forearm rotation at all, but still bleeds into the joint, causing pain and loss of elbow motion. Though the undisplaced fracture may not need surgery, it is just as important that the elbow motion be restored. This means that, after a short period of splinting, the patient has to be encouraged to start actively moving the elbow or it will lose some of its motion. Usually, this means it won't straighten out all the way, or perhaps it won't bend up as far as it should.

For these reasons, the name of the game with elbow fractures is restoring range of motion. If the fracture is

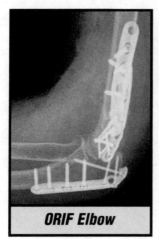

ORIF Elbow

displaced, this may mean fairly extensive surgery with plates, screws and a lot of hardware you just don't want to think about. We call this kind of surgery, "open reduction and internal fixation," or ORIF, for short. This terminology applies to any joint or long bone that we have to open up to fix. Fixation of bad elbow fractures has come a long way in the years I've been doing this procedure, but it still isn't an injury you'd wish on your worst enemy. Unfortunately, these pesky fractures are increasing in frequency as we get busier, go faster and take on more risks in our recreational pursuits.

The way we are wired, the Brain is in charge of protecting itself whenever we fall, and it is perfectly willing to sacrifice any or all of our extremities to do so, even though it's already living in its own heavily fortified ivory tower (the skull). As we topple off that stepladder, the Brain immediately goes into action, sending out emergency orders to the upper extremities to meet the ground first. Since the Brain is the supreme commander, everybody always does whatever it says. In fact, I'm not sure my brain isn't a little miffed right now that I'm giving away its secrets, but that's the way it works. Skull fractures only occur when the body's first line of defenses fail. Even when you fall backward, the Brain throws out your arms, hoping you'll snag *something* and break the fall. Very often, it's the upper extremity joints or long bones that pay this price.

My friend Jim eventually got over his tennis elbow after the surgery and returned to full duty, stamping out spinal disease. And in 1990 it looked like he'd even get his chance to be a war surgeon. About a year after the Western

Hemisphere was made safe for democracy, that old reprobate Saddam Hussein snatched the Kuwaiti oil fields. Like all the other military medical personnel at the time, we were deployed in the Gulf War effort. But once again there was a problem. Our medical center was assigned to staff a huge dormant contingency hospital, pre-positioned in the middle of the English countryside on an abandoned RAF base. Of course, all the war planning had assumed that our enemy would be Russia, not Iraq. This sort of deployment was true for many medics in the Desert Storm campaign. The military just didn't know how many casualties we might have. So they staffed every hospital they had lying in wait all over Europe as well as Southwest Asia. Most went to Saudi Arabia, but many of us went to England, Germany, Spain and Turkey.

In our case off we flew to the Cotswolds, that beautiful area of rolling English hills, thatched houses and sheep. This is the neighborhood of Stratford on Avon, Oxford, Stone Henge, and about as many Iraqis as live in Bozeman, Montana. One of the general surgeons called home and told his wife, "Honey, you could either say this place is pastoral, or bucolic, or in the middle of f**king nowhere." There we hooked up with some 2500 other medics, whereupon we spent the next four months doing absolutely nothing but griping about the boredom and lifting pints in the local pubs. Don't get me wrong; nobody was sorry that we didn't have thousands of wounded soldiers to care for, but you could hardly call us war surgeons for that experience alone. But for all the drinking we did, Jim sure was happy he had a functional elbow.

Chapter 6: The Wrist

One fine day you decide to go out and feed the neighbor's cat while she is on vacation. It seems like an innocent gesture of goodwill, only you put it off until after dark. As you stumble out into the alley in your bathrobe, with your bifocals on and with both hands full of "Nine Lives," you unexpectedly wind up spending one of yours. You trip on the neighbor kid's skateboard and go flying off into the wild blue yonder, scattering the cat food in a great fan of embarrassment. Immediately your brain reaches out to protect itself, throwing both hands out to break the fall. You land with all your weight onto your right wrist. In a split second it shatters into a crooked, excruciating mess that will take months to heal. You have now learned firsthand how crucial the wrist is. It will continue to remind you every time you try to button a blouse, fix your hair, wipe your bottom or type an email. The wrist is like the suburbs of the hand—you drive right through it on the way to the big city and hardly notice it, but, in fact, that's where everybody lives.

Carpal Tunnel Syndrome

Carpal tunnel syndrome may be the most famous orthopedic condition of the modern age. "Carpus" means wrist, so we might as well have called this "wrist tunnel syndrome," but if we didn't have our own mysterious lingo, you might catch on and start treating yourself in your garage. The condition is actually a compressed nerve and has little or nothing to do with the wrist or carpal bones. Though carpal tunnel syndrome affects 3% of Americans—over 8 million people!—it is common to see patients who are referred with this diagnosis, who really have something else. It has gotten to the point where almost anything and everything that hurts anywhere in the general neighborhood of the wrist is attributed to carpal tunnel syndrome.

True carpal tunnel syndrome is a compression of the median nerve, the nerve that passes through the carpal tunnel on its way to the fingers and thumb.

If you look at your own hand with the palm up, the floor of this carpal tunnel is made up of the bones of your wrist. The roof of the tunnel is a strap of ligament (carpal ligament) that spans the distance from the base of the 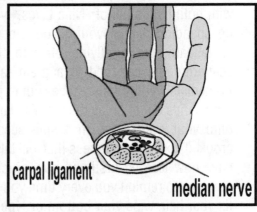 thumb to the base of the small finger side of the palm. Through this canal run all the tendons that bend your fingers and this one darn nerve. The problem here is not the nerve; it's the company it keeps. When positioned at the extremes of flexion or extension, or placed in any sustained posture for a prolonged period of time, the tendons take up most of the available space in the canal and the nerve gets crowded, in other words, pinched. The symptoms of carpal tunnel syndrome are *nerve* symptoms in the areas where the median nerve goes. This means numbness, or tingling in the thumb, index, long and part of the ring fingers and sometimes weakness in the thumb muscles. Patients will typically describe this as the "hand going to sleep," and since this occurs frequently at night, people rarely figure out that the little finger is not affected. "My whole hand goes to sleep, Doc," is the common history. This uncomfortable feeling may be associated with various descriptions of pain, burning, feeling a loss of circulation etc, but the primary feature of carpal tunnel syndrome should always be numbness.

To cloud the issue even more, there can be associated pains anywhere along the path of the median nerve on its way from the neck to the hand. Shoulder pain is common, and sometimes forearm pains and even neck pain. So, you can see that this common problem may have some uncommon presentations, which makes it confusing to get to the bottom of it. Often the doctor will order "nerve conduction studies" to test the way the median nerve conducts electricity along its route. (We've seen these used before at the elbow for ulnar nerve compression.) If the problem is truly carpal tunnel syndrome, there will usually be a slowing of conduction across the wrist.

Once the diagnosis is confirmed, the treatment involves four things: avoidance of the activities that provoke it (have you heard this before?); splinting, particularly at night; cortisone shots to shrink swelling in those pesky neighboring tendons; and, finally, surgery to raise the roof of the tunnel and make more room for the nerve. Libraries of information have been offered about workplace modifications, pressure from keyboards, wrist pads pro and con, and all that. But, once again, we were not designed to sit at a keyboard and hammer away for eight hours a day. If that is what you do for a living, you should just tell your boss that you are going out to cut up a wildebeest or two and that you'll be back in an hour.

Since I see loads of patients with this condition, carpal tunnel release is one of the most common procedures I do. We usually start up that stepladder of treatment options beginning with rest, splinting and injections before we get to surgery, but there are times when we skip right to surgery. These are the cases where there is already a wasting of the thumb muscles where the nerve enters, constant numbness that doesn't go away during the day, or waking up seven out of seven nights with symptoms, despite splinting. Patients often ask me if they are risking "permanent nerve damage" by putting off surgery. The answer is yes, if they wait until they have numbness all day long or weakness in the thumb muscles supplied by the median nerve. As long as they aren't to that stage, I think it's safe to wait and continue with splinting and injections—as long as they are helpful.

The surgery leaves a small scar in the palm, which is tender for several weeks, but usually fades to almost nothing within the first year. I've had patients who have had one side done years ago and neither they nor I can tell which one it was by looking at the palm. Complications include stiffness requiring physical therapy, injury to the nerve at surgery, pain in the palmar scar and recurrence. By this I mean that you can have an excellent surgical result and then eventually get a recurrence by going back to the same work habits or just by further compression of the nerve over time. Surgery is much less successful for those unfortunate patients who find themselves in this situation. Then it's definitely time to find a job hunting wildebeests.

DeQuervain's Tendonitis

Another of the afflictions that affects the wrist is tendonitis. The most common form actually involves the tendons that extend the thumb. The thumb has three bones and three joints. For each of those joints, there is a tendon whose sole job it is to pull on the bone in question, drawing it up and away from the plane of the palm.

Two of these tendons bunk together in one sheath in what I consider another of those little mistakes God made on the

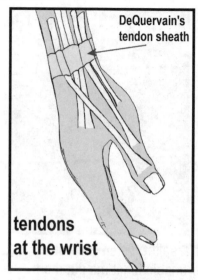

DeQuervain's tendon sheath

tendons at the wrist

last part of Day Six of Creation, just before He rested. Maybe He delegated this design to one of those angels who were later cast out of Paradise. All I know is that this arrangement causes the wrist a lot of trouble.

These two tendons cross over the back of the radius where they are strapped down to it in a very tight sheath. Once this sheath gets inflamed, it causes pain over the back of the wrist, worsened by activities that involve the thumb—and almost all hand activities involve the thumb. This particular tendonitis has an *eponym*, meaning that some lucky doctor went down in history as the first to describe it. Unfortunately for us, it was some French guy named DeQuervain.

The main symptom of DeQuervain's tendonitis is pain during wrist motion felt about where a bracelet or wristwatch would rub on the thumb side of the wrist. Often there is some swelling along the tendon sheath, and in the worst cases there is actually an audible creaking as the tendons move painfully through their sheath. The diagnosis is made by taking a patient's history and giving him or her a fairly simple physical exam that focuses on excluding the other problems that can cause pain in this location. The most common imposter is arthritis in the joint at the base of the thumb. The name of the little test to we do to confirm the diagnosis is even cooler than the name DeQuervain's. It's called the Finkelstein test. This involves having the patient first clasp his thumb inside of his palm, and then flexing his wrist away from the thumb. A positive

Finkelstein's test means either getting punched in the nose by the patient for the excruciating pain this movement elicits, or hearing an agonizing groaning sound, at times accompanied by a ripe expletive.

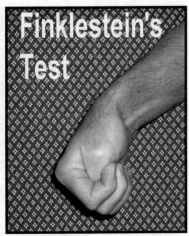

Finklestein's Test

The treatment is a cortisone shot into the tendon sheath, sometimes accompanied by several days of wearing a cast or a splint. Often the patient comes to the first visit unwilling or unable to let me put them in a cast, so we usually compromise and do just the shot. I tell them, though, that if that doesn't do the trick, the next step is to repeat the injection and then add the casting. As always, for the recalcitrant cases the final solution is surgical. Here we simply incise the tendon sheath along its length, freeing up the tendons. Think of it as letting out the pants on a fifty-year-old veteran's war uniform. This is an outpatient procedure done under a local anesthetic with a little sedation. We splint the wrist for about a week post-op, and most people get excellent relief without any residual weakness.

DeQuervain's is one of those overuse conditions that has become much more common with the explosion of computer keyboard usage. In patients who present with a work-related DeQuervain's syndrome, I do the shots and the splinting, but I encourage them to meet with the occupational therapist for a workstation evaluation before considering surgery. If you do surgery for something that is really related to an awkward or inefficient workstation position, or an unrealistic job description, the surgery is doomed to failure. This brings us back to the hunting-the-wildebeest analogy. The human hand

and wrist were just not designed for hammering away day after day at a keyboard, and that can't be remedied surgically.

Intersection Syndrome

There is another less common tendonitis that involves mostly paddling sports, such as canoeing or kayaking. Kathy and I love to canoe and we share this recreational activity with other boomers. Most of us just like to float down a nice creek or paddle around a lake, but there are those among us, usually the risk takers, who push paddling sports to the extreme. These are the dudes who you see going over the falls in a kayak with a big dumb grin on their faces. These are the guys who take off a few weeks to run the Colorado through the Grand Canyon, or maybe recreate Lewis and Clark's expedition by paddling *up* the Missouri River.

There is a crossroads about halfway down the forearm where the tendons that extend the thumb cross over the tendons that extend the wrist. The constant friction that can occur at this site during prolonged paddling may cause an inflammation between these two tendon groups. This is called "Intersection Syndrome." Though there is no true tendon sheath here, this is more like a bursitis in the tissues between these two tendon groups. As with DeQuervain's Syndrome, there is localized pain and often a creaking or "crepitus," as we call it. The treatment is similar to other tendonitis conditions: rest, cortisone injections and splinting. This one almost never needs surgery.

Fractures

The most common wrist fracture occurs when a person falls on his or her outstretched hand. Most of the time, the hand is forced backward and either the small bones of the wrist give or the end of the radius bone cracks.

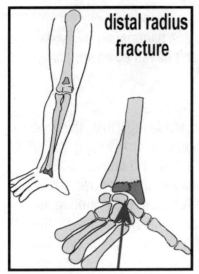

distal radius fracture

I'll deal with fractures of the distal radius first. Recently we saw an epidemic of these wrist fractures from the popular new scooters. Before that it was skateboards. So far it's mostly kids, but give the boomers a few months and they'll be trying out this new fad.

Fractures of the distal radius occur most commonly in older women, since this is generally one of those fractures we associate with osteoporosis, the thinning of the bones with aging. When Grandma falls and her brain automatically tries to protect her body, her hand goes out and the weakest link in the chain is usually the distal end of the radius at the wrist. Some women in midlife already have osteoporosis and can suffer wrist fractures from innocent falls, much like elderly women. We'll discuss osteoporosis in detail in a later chapter.

In most boomers, however, it takes a lot more energy to fracture our healthy bones. So, for us, this is often an injury that happens at high-energy, high-velocity activities, such as motor vehicle calamities and falls from speeding bicycles, jet skis, high ladders etc. In fact, the end of the radius may actually be so sturdy that the same type of injury that would break Granny's radius will instead only fracture one of the smaller bones of the boomer's wrist. Subtle differences in wrist position at the time of impact will also cause a different array of injuries but, suffice it to say, those fractures of the wrist that we see in boomers are a different fish than we see in the elderly.

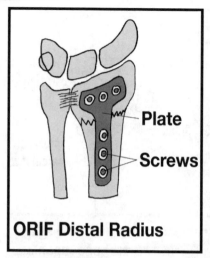

ORIF Distal Radius

Plate

Screws

When boomers do suffer a fracture of the distal radius, the injury tends to be shattered bone with a lot of displacement. For this reason these fractures are less treatable with casting and more often require surgery. Surgery may involve open reduction and internal fixation (known as "ORIF," as we talked about in the shoulder).

ORIF of the radius at the wrist usually involves opening it up, setting the fracture ("reducing" it), often bone grafting it and putting in a plate and screws to hold the broken parts together. Sometimes we use a technique we call "external fixation." With this technique we set the fracture by pulling the bone back out to its full length, and then holding the wrist in that position by what is known as "walking traction." What this means is that we place pins through the skin and into the bone of the hand below the fracture, and then into the radius bone above the fracture. These pins are then attached to a frame apparatus that holds the pins apart at a fixed length.

The whole contraption is left in place until that fracture has healed, and then removed.

Fractures of the small bones of the wrist are also nasty. One in particular, a fracture of the scaphoid bone, is both common and peculiarly bothersome. The way the small bones of the wrists work is very complicated and whole textbooks

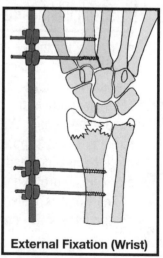

External Fixation (Wrist)

have been written about it. Conferences that last for days and abound with controversy surround this subject. I'm going to try to make it simple, but it is actually a long way from it. There are two rows of small bones in the wrist called the carpal bones. These carpal

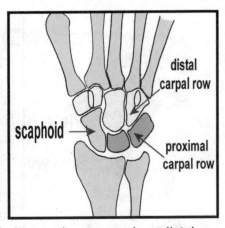

bones fall into a proximal (nearest) row, and a distal (farthest) row. One bone spans both rows and works to coordinate the motions between them.

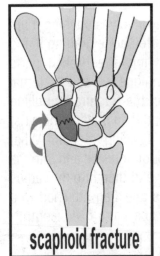

scaphoid fracture

When the wrist is suddenly forced backward beyond its limit, this spanning bone, the scaphoid, breaks in the middle. Basically, one part of it tries to follow the proximal row and the other tries to follow the distal row. It's like being friends with both sides of a divorced couple. Nobody wins. Once fractured, the scaphoid is notorious for either not healing or, even if it heals, going on to soften and collapse. Both of these calamities arise from the same unique disadvantage. The scaphoid is almost completely covered in joint cartilage, living as it does deep inside the wrist. With this arrangement, there is a very tenuous blood supply to this bone that makes it hard for it to mount a healing response. Even if it does, it may heal only to die. This failure to heal is called a "non-union," and the death of the bone is called "osteonecrosis." Both non-union and osteonecrosis are common complications of any bone that has an iffy blood supply, or that lies almost completely within a joint and is covered by articular cartilage. We will encounter this situation several more times. The hip and the ankle are two other bones of this type and therefore common locations for osteonecrosis.

For all these reasons, fractures of the scaphoid are high-risk injuries that can be hard to treat and even harder to diagnose. If the fracture is sustained with a fall on the outstretched hand, the patient may not have any real deformity, but may end up with only a little swelling and limitation of wrist motion, accompanied by pain between the wrist and the base of the thumb, an area we call the "anatomic snuffbox."

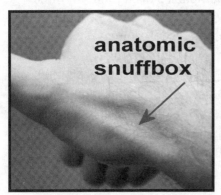

Patients and sometimes doctors often blow these injuries off as a "sprained wrist." We orthopods have a truism: a "sprained wrist" is a fracture of the scaphoid until proven otherwise. Therefore, all painful wrists after a fall should be x-rayed, but even then these little rascals can be hard to see. A hairline crack in the scaphoid may not at first be visible on a plain x-ray. Even sophisticated techniques may miss this injury and the patient can waltz out of the office or the Emergency Room thinking he's out of the woods. Then the pain persists and, down the line, the wrist falls apart. So, the best policy is to cast all these injuries and re-x-ray them in a week. Usually, at this stage there has been some resorption of bone along the fracture line (the first part of the healing process) and the fracture actually becomes easier to see. If at one week the patient still has pain in the anatomic snuffbox, and a negative x-ray, then we either order an MRI or a CT scan. Once again, the risks of missing this diagnosis are so high that this sort of full court press is warranted. An undisplaced fracture of this bone has a ninety plus percent chance of healing without problems if placed in a cast. If not recognized and allowed to displace, the wrist will go to hell in a hand basket.

Not all fractures of this bone are hairline cracks or undisplaced fractures. Those that are displaced require open reduction and either fixation with pins or a small screw designed for just this tricky job. Sometimes boomers with fractures that could be treated in a cast will opt for surgical fixation to get the healing process over with quicker. The prolonged disability that accompanies living up to three months in a cast has pushed doctors toward more aggressive operative treatment of these fractures. Obviously, this is a tradeoff that asks the patient to weigh the risks of surgical intervention against those of prolonged immobilization in a cast and a period of rehabilitation to get the adjacent joints moving again and get rid of the stiffness. As a surgeon, I would probably have mine fixed, but I would offer you both options and help you decide what's best for your situation.

Ganglions

Finally, the wrist is prone to a particular type of swelling that we call a ganglion cyst. These cysts arise from the joint itself and always communicate with it. They are filled with a fluid that is something like joint fluid, though thicker. Originally, the theory was that these swellings were little bulges from the joint that pooched out at weak points and got filled with

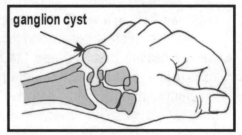

ganglion cyst

the joint's own fluid, which then became concentrated or thickened. This is probably only partly correct and, like so many other things, we actually don't completely understand where these ganglions come from or why. They typically fluctuate in size and, at first, are usually not that painful. After a time, however, they may get large enough to either cause pain or to crowd the adjacent tendons. Sometimes, they are just cosmetically unsightly, but more often the patient experiences a combination of pain, anxiety over what this growth really is, and concern about its unattractive appearance.

The most common location for these ganglions is on the back of the wrist. Here they are easier to treat, as they always come from the same location, from one ligament between the same two bones. There are two treatments and one folk remedy. The folk remedy is to smash the ganglion with a large book, preferably a Bible. This seems to work in some patients, and I've seen quite a number through the years who confess to having either tried it or contemplated it. The two treatments recommended by doctors are to stick a needle into the ganglion after numbing it, suck out the fluid and then put in a drop of cortisone. Some doctors skip the cortisone. I usually add a week of splinting or casting, because the way this procedure is supposed to work is by scarring up the stalk at the base of the ganglion where it communicates with the joint. Scarring is more likely to occur if the wrist is not moving. This procedure is reported to work as often as eighty percent of the time, though my personal experience has shown me that it works less often than that. I still always offer this as the first treatment, at least for ganglions on the backside of the wrist.

The surgical treatment is to cut the darn thing out, which means an operation that goes down to the joint and removes the source of the problem. This trades in a bump for a small scar and has about a one in twenty recurrence rate.

Ganglions on the palm side of the wrist are more difficult to treat. Here they can arise from at least two, and probably three different places, so the surgeon can't be quite as certain that he's gotten to the source of the cyst. Add to this that these palmar wrist ganglions bubble up between the artery to the hand and adjacent nerves, so the stakes in treating them successfully get a little higher. The recurrence rate is a little more frequent, and the surgery is a little trickier. Nevertheless, for the hand surgeon and most general orthopedists, it's just another day at the office.

And this brings me to a word or two about whom you should allow to operate on your wrist or hand. Most hand surgeons[7] are orthopedists, but not all orthopedists are hand surgeons. Other doctors who operate on the hand include a few well-trained plastic surgeons and a very few general surgeons. There isn't a lot of room for avoiding screw-ups where so many vital functions are packed so tightly together. So you want to know something about the training and experience of the doc who wants to operate on you.

Tendonitis, fractures of various kinds, ganglion cysts—there are many ways that the wrist can slow down a boomer. In general, these conditions all arise from some combination of overuse, misjudgment and/or genetic predisposition. Some people have tighter tendon sheaths than others. Some have riskier jobs or jobs that simply ask way too much of the wrist. About all you can do to avoid these problems is watch out for skateboards when you go out to feed that neighbor's cat. I would *never* go up on a ladder without a spotter and I wouldn't walk down a stairway without turning on the lights, no matter how familiar I was with the territory. I can't afford to be out for three months with a broken scaphoid. Can you?

---

7 "Hand surgeons" generally operate on most upper extremity problems, but especially wrist and hand.

Chapter 7: The Hand

Early in my career I thought I wanted to be a hand surgeon. In fact, I started my residency thinking I was probably going to specialize exclusively in the hand. My advisor in medical school at the University of Iowa was a world famous hand surgeon, Dr. Adrian Flatt. An Englishman and a former WWII British flight surgeon who had grown up in India, he was in all ways larger than life. He took me under his wing, and as a medical student, I got to train with him twice. It was he who advised me to leave Iowa City and pursue my training at Mayo's, lest I become "provincial," as he put it, by spending kindergarten through residency all in Iowa City.

At Mayo's I trained with two other world famous hand surgeons, Dr. Ron Lindscheid and Dr. Jim Dobyns. I also did six months of microvascular research at a time when this was all brand new stuff. We essentially taught ourselves how to sew together two-millimeter blood vessels under the microscope, using some clues we'd gotten from the Chinese and a few other American surgical pioneers.

Along the way I was also exposed to all the other wonderful things exploding onto the orthopedic scene in those days, especially total joint replacement and arthroscopy. I eventually realized that I was fascinated with too many other things to narrow my practice to just hands. But I've never lost my interest in this crown jewel of all surgical specialties, and hand surgery is still a large and very gratifying part of my practice.

The hand is the most commonly injured part of the body, as long as you don't count pride. There is still some debate among anthropologists and anatomists as to whether the brain increased in size because of the added demands placed on it by the ever-evolving hands, once we went bipedal. If you look at the amount of brain devoted to various parts of the body, as in this famous depiction of the "homunculus," you can see the fondness that the boss has for his workers, the hands, and especially the thumb. A disproportionate amount of the sensory part of the brain is devoted to the thumb. In Tom Robbins' wonderful book *Even Cowgirls Get the Blues* the heroine has these great outsized thumbs. I've always wondered if Robbins had seen this homunculus, or just intuited this bit of anatomic favoritism.

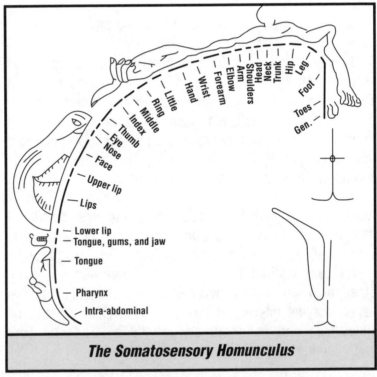

The Somatosensory Homunculus

The hand is wonderfully complicated. And yet it is a remarkable design of mobility, strength, sensitivity, quickness and beauty. The same hand that can play Mozart can club that wildebeest. On the same day, it can touch you with such subtlety that you quiver with delight, or it can just as easily break your nose. Do you remember what is was like the last time you had a hand injury, even a little cut finger? All it takes is one small ding and you suddenly recognize how much you've been taking this guy for granted. Everybody's had that finger caught in the car door, that smashed nail, or that sprained middle joint from playing basketball and catching it right on the end of the finger. Not only does the injury hurt like crazy, but there's the dysfunction it causes the whole hand, not to mention the compensation and reordering necessary to cope with losing this or that player from the lineup.

I'll discuss the injuries and maladies of the soft parts first: tendonitis, bumps and catches, tendon lacerations and cutaneous injuries. Then I'll go over the bone and joint injuries and afflictions: fractures, dislocations and arthritis.

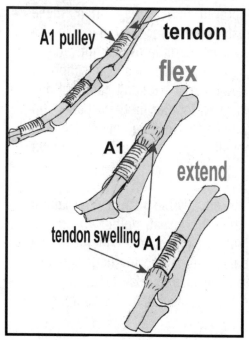

Trigger Finger

Here's an easy malady to visualize, the "trigger finger." It sounds like what it is, a painful catching of the tendon that flexes your finger. In this condition the tendon gets swollen and catches up on one of the first tunnels it passes through on its way to work.

This particular tunnel, which we doctors call

the A1 pulley or "first annular pulley," is deep within the palm where the tendon is strapped down to the metacarpal bone.

This condition can affect any digit, including the thumb, in which case it gets called "trigger thumb." See, I told you this was easy. The catching arises from some inflammation along the tendon sheath, sometimes caused by simple overuse, such as a lot of tool gripping or lifting narrow-handled buckets. It also can be related to those many conditions that cause inflammation, including rheumatoid arthritis, lupus, diabetes or thyroid conditions. Most of the time, however, neither the patient nor the doctor has a clue where this problem comes from.

Patients usually just describe a painful catching of the finger. They may recognize that the source is in the palm, but just as often they relate the catching to the middle joint of the finger, which seems to lock. It may take some persuasion to convince the patient that the cause is down there in the palm, when the effect is up here in finger. Very often, these triggering fingers are most bothersome first thing in the morning. The hand always swells a little over night, due to inactivity, and sometimes from the venous congestion of sleeping on that arm. A tendon that wouldn't catch all day after it's "warmed up" will snap for the first few hand grip cycles, usually limbering up after making the coffee and shaving. (At least that's how it works in the case of my own middle finger).

If the triggering never gets any worse than a few painful startups in the morning, then, no sweat, nothing needs be done. Most of those patients never get bad enough to see me. But if it becomes a daily routine and the finger gets to where it catches any time it pleases, all day long, then it's time for treatment. Since this is ultimately a tendonitis or inflammation of the tendon in its sheath, it can often be reversed with a cortisone shot. Once the condition has been around long enough for some of the inflammatory tissue to become thickened and fibrotic (as we call it), then a shot alone won't help. In the cases that fail to respond to a shot or two, we move rather quickly to surgical release of the pulley. Like many other procedures in the hand, this can be done as an outpatient under local anesthetic. In fact, it is literally a ten-minute, two-stitch job. It is not unusual to do two or three fingers either at the same time or over a period of time for one patient.

The patients that I see probably get this most often from home building projects, office work with repetitive hand maneuvers, home crafts and hobbies, and a few from bicycling. The grip position for mountain biking seems particularly irritating to some people who may be prone to this condition.

Tendon Lacerations

Though tendonitis can be annoying, cutting a tendon is as serious as taxes. To cut the extensor tendons on the back of the wrist or fingers is bad enough, but to slice a flexor tendon on the palm side of a finger is very serious business. We call these injuries "flexor tendon lacerations," and they are bad news, worse than injuries to the tendons that extend the fingers. The same principles of treatment and prevention apply to extensor tendon injuries as well, but, in general, it's easier on both the patient and the hand surgeon to get a good result on the back of the hand.

Cut up the business side of the hand, and the Brain doesn't like it. It immediately sends out commands to the other hand and even the adjacent digits to stem the bleeding, hold the damaged thing still and fumble through the phone book for the nearest hand surgeon.

Flexor tendon lacerations most often occur in the kitchen or the other places humans use knives to cut things: fishing, hunting, hobby-ing, camping etc. We get lazy; we lose respect for that sharp object we're wielding with such aplomb. "Do this every day, man. Cut those carrots first, then the peppers and then the… OUCH! Damn, that's a deep one this time, you idiot. Shit, will you look at that! I can't even move the damn thing. Must have cut a tendon! Think I'll sit down. Where's that phone book?" When you seriously injure yourself, you experience all the classic stages of grief: denial, anger, remorse, resignation. You can go through all those stages, but you need to get through them as quickly as possible, because the damage is done. Though people often get excellent results from the way we repair and rehabilitate flexor tendon lacerations today, it is just as likely that a person may experience some residual loss of motion, flexibility, dexterity or strength. It's clearly better just not to cut the darn things in the first place. And here we *can be* more careful, as these injuries are essentially the equivalent of an LAE for the hand.

Don't do risky things with your hands. Please cut *away* from the hand not toward it. That move your grandmother did with the little paring knife cupped in the palm, the blade up toward the thumb, slicing the potato or the carrot against the thumb—that move is very dangerous. Use a cutting board and cut away from yourself. Better yet, use a machine to do the job. Avoid using "knife" and "slimy thing" in the same sentence. Every year at Halloween doctors see plenty of victims of pumpkin carving. Slippery buggers those pumpkins. You mark out your design for the old jacko-lantern with Magic Marker and then you pop the top on the big squash. Now things start to go sour. You start digging out the innards; all the slimy seeds in the slimy little squashy stringy stuff. If you are smart, then and *only then* do you pick up the knife. If you start trying to slice all that stuff out, you have a classic recipe for disaster. You could substitute "mango" or even "avocado" for the pumpkin and you would have the same constellation of factors that puts the hand at great risk.

Once cut, the flexor tendon needs to be repaired. I suppose that sounds easy and it would be, were it not for two very big obstacles. First, for almost the whole length of the finger, the tendon glides through a smooth tube, and within this tube the tolerances are very small. No room for sutures; no room for scarring. Second, while it would be nice not to move the tendon to allow it to heal properly, not moving it while it's healing guarantees it will never move again. This combination of challenges forces us into a rob-Peter-to-pay-Paul situation. You have no choice but to fix it and move it both. Up until well after WWII, flexor tendon lacerations in the mid finger, the so-called "No Man's Land," were simply not repaired initially following an injury. The results of operating in this tight spot were just too lousy. Instead, the tendons were left unsutured, while the finger was prepared for the inevitable tendon transfer.

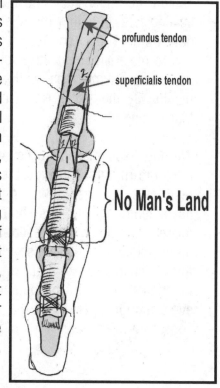

profundus tendon

superficialis tendon

No Man's Land

After the tendon had "died," it was replaced with a free tendon graft or transfer. In other words, no one dared go into No Man's Land and risk a primary repair of the tendon. The resultant scarring and stiffness made the end result worse than no operation.

In the 1960s a few brave souls began opening the lacerated tendon sheath, and gently and carefully repairing the tendon with stitches that would hold firmly enough so that the finger could be moved right away. They worked out an ingenious splint that would allow the patient to move the finger without using the repaired tendon. This crafty "dynamic splint" allowed the patient to actively straighten the finger in a controlled fashion, moving the tendon within the sheath and minimizing scarring. A strategically placed rubber band would then substitute for the damaged tendon's function, pulling the finger back into flexion, once again moving the healing tendon within the sheath. This combination of the development of new less traumatic techniques, better suture materials, innovative rehabilitation schemes and the courage to attempt repair in this area led to surprisingly good results. By the 1970s No Man's Land had become "Some Man's Land."

We now expect lacerated flexor tendons to heal with a low rate of re-rupture, and expect to get very good, if not perfect, restoration of finger motion. And we now feel that most such flexor tendon lacerations should be repaired surgically and moved right away. The patient might have a hand that's tied up in splinting for at least six weeks and tied up with therapy for at least three to four months. But he can expect a functional finger, capable of doing most of what it used to do, even though there may be some limitation of motion compared to normal.

Bumps and Lumps

Coming as it does so often into harm's way, the hand is prone to lumps and bumps. The three most common masses in the hand—ganglion cysts, epidermal inclusion cysts, and the little rascal called "the giant cell tumor of tendon sheath"—can all safely be removed with a low recurrence rate. Though these lumps all have their distinguishing characteristics, sometimes you're not sure what it is until you take it out and biopsy it. All the big three have very distinct appearances on the operating table, so most of the time if we're not already pretty sure what it is, we're going to know as soon as we're removing it. There can be a host of other things lurking around the hand, but the numbers are so small that they can be considered negligible. But this shouldn't lead the casual hand surgeon into complacency. Every now and then a benign appearing lump turns out to be something with very serious ramifications. We are only occasionally surprised by the biopsy diagnosis, but we should be careful to warn our patients that almost any lump can be serious, and the only way to really be sure is to remove it and biopsy it.

I had a very recent reminder of this principle and though the lump in question was actually at the elbow, it illustrates this point vividly. I saw a patient in the clinic for a knee problem and he asked me incidentally about a lump he had on the inside of his elbow. He said that he'd had it at least three years, it hadn't grown much and it was more or less just a nuisance. It didn't hurt, but he wondered what I thought it was. He added that his father, a senior general surgeon, had told him not to worry about it. It was about the size of a small grape, the skin over it was freely mobile (a good sign in that many malignancies grab the skin above them), non-tender and in all ways appeared benign. I said, "Well, the only way to know what this is, is to take it out and biopsy it. If it looks funky, I'll do a frozen section, but if it looks benign, we'll just excise it and send it in." At surgery a month or so later, it looked benign enough that I simply excised it and some of the surrounding soft tissue, sent it in and reassured the patient and his wife. Just before I saw him back in the clinic a few days later, the biopsy report was still not available. I called the pathologist to get the report and he told me that it was a very rare, high-grade malignancy, something so rare that they'd sent it off to several other even larger labs for confirmation. I had to walk into the room and tell the patient that I was not only wrong, but possibly dead wrong.

You recall, ganglion cysts occur at the wrist joint and may occur on either the back or the palmar. There is one particular variation on the ganglion theme that occurs in the fingers and palms of the boomer age group. A small ganglion cyst will bubble up on the palmar side of the finger or in the palm near the crease. These ganglions, which are associated with the tendon sheath, are called "retinacular cysts" for reasons lost to antiquity. These are usually painful enough to require either aspiration with a needle or surgical removal. Like all ganglions, they can fluctuate in size. Lying as they do along the major trade routes of the hand, the Brain often sends priority mail messages about these ganglions. "Get rid of that little painful thing in my finger will ya'? Yesterday would be soon enough!"

Epidermal inclusion cysts are actually cystic tumors that arise from skin cells being inoculated under the skin. Sometimes a laceration or a deep poke will trap some of the superficial skin cells deep under the skin. There they continue to produce the protective layer of keratin that would normally get washed or abraded away with daily use. This keratin collects in a cyst and slowly enlarges. It may even cause enough pressure to erode into the adjacent bones. These lumps are painful only when they grow large enough to push around the adjacent structures. At surgery they are filled with what looks like cream cheese—they are very distinctive and easy to recognize.

So-called "giant cell tumor of tendon sheath" is a bad name in a lot of ways, but it sounds worse than it is. It's a fibrous lump that forms, usually in the finger and though it may recur after removal, is benign and self-limiting. I mention it here in case your doctor shocks you by telling you that "GCT is in the differential diagnosis" of that lump in your hand. It sounds awful, but it's just another benign soft-tissue tumor with an ugly name.

Little fatty tumors, lipomas, do occur around the hand but are diagnosed far too often when the real culprit is one of the big three. This is also a favorite diagnosis of general surgeons who wander unexpectedly into hand surgery. Lipomas are nowhere near as common in the hand as elsewhere in the body where we usually find them, typically on the trunk and proximal limbs.

Metastatic cancers occur so infrequently in the hand that they too lull us into not expecting them to happen at all. I once had a patient whom I'd treated previously for a metastatic breast cancer that had caused a hip fracture. We'd gotten her through that with a fancy hip replacement prosthesis that had allowed me to cut the cancer out with the bone. Now, a year or more later, she had a swelling on her wrist. Her oncologist sent her to me for this "ganglion." The x-ray showed complete destruction of the end of the radius from the metastatic cancer that had come marching up out of the bone and up under the skin over the wrist. So, it does happen, but not very often.

Dupuytren's Contracture

I have a hard time explaining this one to patients, even when it's sitting right there in front of both of us. This condition is more common with aging, but I've seen some boomers developing this in their mid fifties. "Contracture" is the business end of this condition, describing a band of thick fibrous tissue that grows from the palm's own ligaments and then slowly thickens and shortens, pulling the poor finger along with it. Dupuytren was the 18th Century French surgeon who finally pointed out that this was not something to do with the tendons. He discovered that this contracting band was made up not of tumor cells, but of a weird kind of thick fibrous tissue superficial to the tendon. Lying beneath this tangled cord that was strangling its precious finger, the tendon was fine. He and others discovered that you could either cut the cord for some minor improvement or even go for the whole enchilada and remove it completely. This problem is more common in Celtic races and more common in alcoholics (am I being redundant here?). Well, you can't do much about being Irish, I can vouch for that. But you can stop abusing the beverage, though that alone won't affect the Dupuytren's.

The surgical treatment for this today involves complete removal of the Dupuytren's cord of contracted tissue, without removing any of the other vital structures concentrated in this area. These things get tangled up with the small nerves that go to the individual sides of the fingers. Damaging these digital nerves or the tendon that lies directly under the diseased tissue is the biggest risk. Because in this condition the fibrous cord actually adheres to the skin, there is also a risk that the skin will not heal so well after being stripped of the damage. The skin has also shortened with the contracting finger, so fancy skin flaps and even skin grafting are sometimes required to get skin coverage over the area where the cord was excised. As with most hand surgeries of any magnitude, the patient can count on at least four to six weeks of splinting and up to three months of therapy to get the hand moving.

Nail Injuries

I'm going to leave alone all the dietary deficiencies, obscure diseases and infestations that can present as changes in the human fingernail. The most astute diagnosticians can look at nail changes and see various pulmonary conditions, vitamin deficiencies, fungal conditions etc. In my office I most commonly see injuries to the nail end of the finger. Most are self-inflicted injuries sustained while working with things that come together forcefully or cut. Things that come together quickly, unexpectedly and sharply are especially well suited to cause injuries to the very tip of the finger just as it's fleeing the scene of the disaster. Fingertips get caught in doors and drawers, cut with snips and paper cutters, and trimmed with carpet tools and a whole grisly arsenal of power-driven, belt-sanding, finger-whacking stuff. The Home Depot from hell. We deliver!

These nail injuries fall into two basic categories. One involves injuries to the nail plate; the other involves injuries to the nail bed from which the plate grows. Injuries to just the nail plate, including those in which the nail gets raised back and avulsed from its bed,

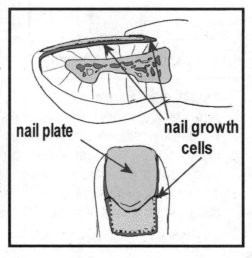

nail plate

nail growth cells

usually heal without much in the way of residuals. While these injuries can be incredibly painful, just keeping the nail plate in place as a splint is about all that's needed for success. But the underlying nail bed and the soft tissue from which the nail plate is made—the nail plate factory, if you will—does not respond as well to injury.

The simplest nail plate injury is an acute bleeding that can occur when the nail is smashed down, squishing the soft nail bed between the hard nail plate and the even harder bone below. The nail bed gets bruised and raises a collection of blood under the nail under extreme pressure. These "subungual hematomas" hurt like crazy. There may even be an underlying fracture of the bone, but even that wouldn't hurt as much as a subungual hematoma that needs to be drained.

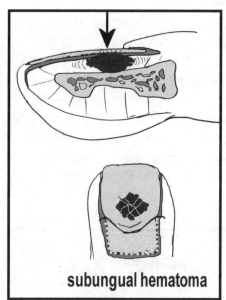

subungual hematoma

These sometimes play out as real heroic ER episodes where the patient comes running in from working on that swing set he was building for Brandon. He's holding his fat, bloody thumb out like it's a dead baby. He's sweating, full of remorse, and in great pain. In walks the brave hand surgeon. He quickly assesses the situation and asks calmly, with a steady voice, "Ya'll got a paperclip? Thanks, Darlin'.[8] Now who's got a BIC lighter? Great... everybody stand back." Then he un-bends the paper clip into a little figure four, flames one end of it with the BIC, and when it's Allentown hot

8 For those of you who would consider this a sexist, demeaning way to talk to a woman, well, you're probably right, but that's how everyone talks to each other in New Orleans. You drive into the Burger King and the gal on the horn says, "Hey, Sugar, what d'ya want?"

he plunges it steaming into the middle of the nail. Bull's-eye! A little puff of steam as the paperclip vaporizes its hole through the nail and the old blood of the hematoma comes erupting out. The patient gets immediate, complete, orgasmic, hug-the-doctor relief. Of course, you can do this with high tech gear like electrocautery units. But you know something? We use the old paperclip trick for the same reason that we make the nurse go get a metal basin when we take a bullet out of someone. The plastic ones just *don't sound right* for a DHP. That's short for a "Doc Holiday Procedure."

Other injuries to the nail bed are not so easy to treat as subungual hematomas. Crushing and slicing injuries that breach the defense of the rigid nail plate and hit the vulnerable nail bed may cause permanent nail deformity. For that reason, we feel that most nail bed injuries should be cleaned up and repaired, often with microscopic sutures. Then either the original nail plate, if is available, or some substitute like plastic or rubber should be placed over the nail bed to protect and direct its healing. The name of the game is to get the nail bed to heal with a minimum of scarring since scarring means deformity when the nail later tries to grow out over what was once a smooth surface. The fewer moguls, the better. Unfortunately, most serious nail bed injuries do cause some scarring and may alter nail behavior. It may grow out crooked or only incompletely. The worst that can happen is a nail that grows out painfully because it gets caught up in the scarred nail bed and is never able to keep growing without getting into this constant detour. Here the only reasonable treatment is to give up on the nail, excising it and the cells from whence it came. These nail "ablations" are tricky and, try as we might, nail remnants can get left behind and come back to haunt the patient and surgeon. Still having no nail on one finger and getting rid of what was a painful deformity is a reasonable tradeoff.

Infections Around the Nail

The human fingernail is one of those bodily gifts that can give more than its intended function if you will let it. By this I mean that people in various cultures have found infinite ways of coloring it, curving it, cutting it long, short or otherwise. It even has a place as one of the human sexual signals. Men have short fingernails so they can hunt and catch the wildebeests. Woman have long useless nails so men can feel like they're providing so well for their women that these women don't even have to use their hands. "Couldn't use them if we tried. Lookie here at these nails!" I was involved in a fascinating illustration of this phenomenon on a plane flight recently. I was flying up from New Orleans to Detroit and my standby ticket put me in between two fifty-ish women who were traveling together. I think they were a little new to air travel and I had the pleasure of showing off my worldliness by finding the little table that pulls up out of the armrest (not intuitively obvious), and eventually explaining that in dire cases, just walking up to the john in first class is not a punishable offense. I think all stewardesses like to pair anxious faces and restrooms as directly as possible. The woman on my right in the window seat was wearing long glue-on, decorative to the max, killer nails. I mean the kind with little sparkles and sometimes even messages and script. When the breakfast "snack" arrived, there was one of those little milk cartons. It may well be that Cheerios with milk are boring, but Cheerios without milk are inedible. I had a little trouble getting mine open and hell, I'm a surgeon! When I glanced over, I saw my row mate locked in mortal combat with the little blue and white devil. Fresh Farms, my ass! I'm gonna rip your throat out! Click click click. I sallied forth and heroically wrenched open the little nuisance and we all slurped our Cheerios. Later I watched as she brought out her not insubstantial pocketbook. It had a pretty big zipper and she went after that with two of her appendages, looking a lot like Edward Scissorhands. I just stayed out of the way.

If we'll put up with that in the name of decoration, surely we set some unusual standards for nail health and maybe for nail behavior. Just drive down the street or, better yet, walk the Mall and count the establishments devoted to nail maintenance and decoration. All this nail manipulation can eventually lead to a breakdown in the nail's natural defenses against infection. One part of the standard professional manicure, the technique of cuticle bashing, is to blame for some infections around the nail. The most common of these is called a paronychia. Here an infection gets started under the skin at the base of the nail and usually along one side.

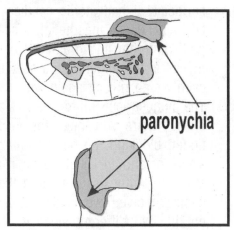

The infection lifts the soft skin up as the pus advances along the soft side of the nail. These throb and hurt a great deal, since the concentration of nerve endings here is among the highest in the body. Paronychias are treated by drainage of the pus, usually an office procedure done under a local anesthetic, and antibiotics. One word of advice, however: make sure the doctor cultures the pus he drains, to discover exactly what bug is causing the infection. Though most of these are the common staphylococcal infections, I've seen examples of almost every bug under the sun. Nobody wants to guess where any given finger has been. I don't even want to know. But I do want to get the antibiotic right.

Not all these nail infections can be blamed on manicurists or their victims. In fact, sometimes it is the exact opposite: poor hygiene or repeated minor injury in the face of an unclean environment. Several years ago I was solo backpacking in the backcountry of Glacier National Park when I developed a painful nail. I watched it evolve into a throbbing, red, swollen paronychia over a few days. When I got out of the woods and back to the bed-and-breakfast where I was staying between hikes, I had everything with me that one needs to deal with it surgically. I had sterile needles and syringes to inject the lidocaine (local anesthetic), a scalpel to lance it, antibiotics both ointment and oral. All I needed was the guts to stab myself in the finger with a needle, inject the drug, and then calmly stab myself again with the blade to let the pus out. The biggest decision for me was actually should I do a finger block, where you inject the local in at the bottom of the finger, blocking the nerves and putting the whole thing to sleep, or should I just go for it and inject directly into the already painful tissue around the fingernail. Since the first choice involved two needle sticks (one for each of the nerves on the two different sides of the finger) and the second choice involved only one shot, I chose door number two.

So here I am in the communal bathroom of this cozy little B&B, whipping out my needles and syringes, drawing up the drug, injecting it, cutting my finger open, bleeding all over the place and then trying to clean it all up as if I had just been in there having a little shave, not some junkie whose heroin shoot went haywire. In the end the relief of releasing pus under pressure is its own reward and after all, I was only a few days from having to go back to operating on people, something you just shouldn't do with pus in your finger.

Sometimes paronychias become quite serious when the infection spreads from the area around the nail and into the pulp of the fingertip. These infections have one of the most appropriate names in all of medicine. They are called "felons." And felonious they are, with the potential to infect the bone and even result in amputation. These occur most commonly in patients with poor immune systems and as we see more such patients these days, we also see more felons. They are also treated by incision, drainage and antibiotics but these more serious infections should be treated in the operating room and not the office (or the john in some B&B in Columbia Falls, Montana).

Fractures and Dislocations

If you don't think baby boomers fracture and dislocate their hands, take a closer look at some of your sports stars. Look at Larry Byrd's index finger or Roger Staubach's pinky. Look at almost any professional basketball player's middle finger joints for the telltale signs of repeated dislocations. How many NBA players have how many taped fingers during any given game? Just translate that to the backyard and playground hoops, throw in softball, flag football, volleyball and rugby, and now multiply it by all the gyms in every town that has one and every softball diamond with or without grass, and you have a lot of busted hands and fingers. You can break any bone or bones in any combination, and the hand has a lot to choose from: five metacarpals and fourteen phalanges. I'll confine my discussion to the most common ones I see in the office. We'll take the dislocations first.

If you look at your own finger, there are three joints. One is at the end (the distal joint), one is in the middle (the proximal joint) and one is where the finger sprouts from the hand (the metacarpopahlangeal joint). Dislocations occur most commonly at the middle joint. Hand surgeons avoid numbering the fingers in order to avoid fistfights over whether the thumb is a finger (in which case it would be the *first* finger), or not a finger (in which case the index would be the first finger). To sidestep this enmity we designate the fingers by names: thumb, index, middle, ring and small. Even whether to call the central digit the "long" or the "middle" spurs debate. Being the most forward it also is among the most commonly injured and often ends up shorter than it started, relinquishing its right to the designation "long."

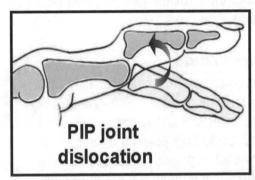

**PIP joint
dislocation**

The common dislocation is of the middle joint of any finger. This frequently occurs to the long or ring fingers. Something hits the already extended finger, forcing it backward at the middle joint until the ligaments finally tear and the bones go "out of joint." The finger looks shortened, the middle bone is riding over the first finger bone and the thing just looks wrong.

Then when the Brain gets wind of this, it sends out an immediate distress, calling for someone to put the joint back in place. The Brain may even take things into its own hands (so to speak) and just give it a good tug with the other hand. This often works as the injured party just pulls on the shortened crooked finger. That maneuver's enough to reduce the dislocation. In the first few minutes after one of these dislocations, it can be popped back in place by the owner or by almost any bystander who doesn't faint while watching *ER*. After only a few golden minutes, however, this protective analgesia rapidly fades. The pain gets slowly worse, until, eventually, the joint can't be reduced unless the finger is put to sleep with a local anesthetic nerve block. Once back in place, these dislocations are usually stable and can be taped to the adjacent finger in a sort of sack race where the healthy leads the lame around for a week or two while the lame is healing.

This same mechanism of injury, when combined with a little more force or velocity, can both dislocate the joint and fracture the bone at the same time. Most of these fractures are only small chips that represent little more than an avulsion of a sliver of bone attached to the ligament that has ruptured. Rather than tear through the ligament, the ligament pulls away from the bone with a little telltale flake of bone from its origin. Even large chip fractures are treated much like ligament sprains: buddy-taping and early motion. Larger fractures may render the joint unstable so that it needs to be reduced, but won't stay that way. In these cases, surgery is necessary to pin or screw the bone back together.

When it comes to fractures, the hand presents a lot of targets. But, unfortunately, it's also commonly aimed at an even greater number of targets. The most common fracture in the hand is the so-called "boxer's fracture," a fracture of the neck of the 5th or small finger metacarpal,

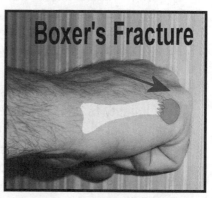

Boxer's Fracture

sustained while wailing away at an unfair world. Unlike in the movies, where you can strike your clenched fist against someone's skull without injury, in real life the fist loses every time. And guess why? Of course, the Brain lives there! The skull is much harder than the hand. Paper covers rock, scissors cut paper, but skull breaks hand every time. And it doesn't even have to be the skull. Wall breaks hand, door breaks hand, locker breaks hand. Hand never breaks wall. Nope, that only happens in the movies.

This simple lesson is repeated day after day, the world over. Somewhere some yak herder is sorry he punched that big hard yak. "What was I thinking? I knew that yak was hard. Hell, they're hard as rocks." I had three offenders in my clinic one afternoon. We had them stacked up "like cord wood," they would say in Minnesota. It is well known among practitioners of the bone-setting art, that a man with a fracture of the neck of the fifth metacarpal, will never, ever tell you the truth, the whole truth or anything like the truth as to how this occurred. I don't even care how he did it, but I love to collect the answers. Like, "Oh, well, I was working in my garage and I fell against an anvil." Or, "Yeah, well, I was on my way to Bible study and I tripped on a Communion wafer." Yeah, right. On that afternoon the only one who gave an even credible story was the boomer lawyer who was moving his office and got pissed at a filing cabinet. The counselor duked out a filing cabinet! Not a brainy move and he knew it, but at least he fessed up.

In fact this is such a brainless move that one wonders where the Almighty Brain is at a time like this. I think what happens here is that the hand can move even faster than certain rational parts of the Brain. It's like the Brain is the parent and the hand is the toddler, running all over, only to be pulled back from the brink of disaster by the seat of his pants. Most of the time, the hand is the servant of the very wishes of the Brain and will respond rapidly on the Brain's behalf in reaction to even deeply disguised passions. I have a feeling that many an about-to-be boxer's fracture is in fact called back on the brink of impact. Sometimes the Brain kicks in just in time. But other times the Brain doesn't recall its own ambassador.

Once the bone is fractured, it angles down a little bit, causing a slight depression of the last knuckle. Though you can make these prettier surgically with pins and or plates and screws, this is usually overkill. Left almost untreated, these do fine. They heal with a barely noticeable deformity and cause little or no functional problems for the hand. This is not to mention that you usually are looking at a somewhat repentant, at least remorseful guy who doesn't really want the world to focus that much on what he's foolishly done to his perfectly good hand. A cast you can laugh off. A trip to the operating room is just a little too much for learning a little about Newton's second law. Rock breaks hand. Hand goes in cast for a few weeks, then fingers taped together for a while, plus-minus a little trip to the physical terrorist, and you're good as new. Or good enough.

Fractures of the other metacarpals are a bit more serious. The way the hand is built, it has a solid central section with the index and long finger metacarpals as the rigid central tent poles. Then it has two mobile borders: the thumb roams around on the one side and the small finger side moves a little bit itself. You can demonstrate this yourself by moving first the fifth and then the fourth metacarpals up and down, toward and away from the palm. They are mobile at their junction with the bones of the wrist. Now try the index and long finger metacarpals. No joy, they are rigidly fixed, anchored solid to their adjacent wrist bones. Because the fourth metacarpal has the motion it has, the fracture can be allowed to angle a little. Though the knuckle is depressed a little bit into the palm, because the metacarpal can move out of the way during grip, this causes little or no problem. If you fracture the long finger metacarpal, however, it can't get out of the way. Any angulation in the long or index finger

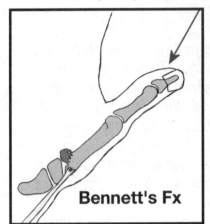

Bennett's Fx

metacarpals is poorly tolerated. For this reason we pin most displaced fractures of these two inboard metacarpals.

At the base of the thumb is a very mobile joint we call the "carpo-meta-carpal" joint. It is one of the sloppiest, most mobile joints in the body, ranking right up there next to the shoulder. When the thumb metacarpal is forced out or the thumb is pushed back, the base of the metacarpal may fracture in a pattern given the eponym "Bennett's fracture." Since this is a fracture into a joint, it deserves an operation to pin it and restore joint congruity.

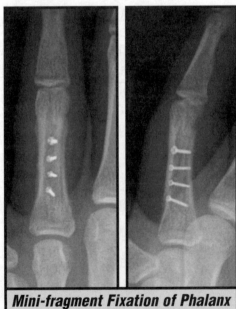

Mini-fragment Fixation of Phalanx Fracture with 1.7mm Screws

Most finger fractures go quickly out of place and need some kind of surgery, either pinning or the newest treatment, tiny screws and plates. Early recognition that you have a problem plays an important role here. I see a lot of people a week or two after their injury. Many times, the patient just thought his or her finger was "jammed" or "sprained" when, in fact, it was broken. The old saw, "I knew it wasn't broke, 'cause I could move it," is just not true. The hand will heal most injuries in some fashion. It will go merrily along and be well along the road to healing a crooked finger by the third week after the calamity. An x-ray is a great test, but it can't help you much if you don't get one done.

The one fracture that is remarkably benign is the fracture of the last "tuft" of the finger's last phalanx. These are usually crush injuries, often caused by pinching or hammering. They may be associated with the infamous nail hematoma, or even injuries to the nail and nail bed. As long as the nail plate is intact over the tuft fracture, it will heal just fine. If the nail is gone, some nail substitute should be used or one should even consider pinning the fracture for a few weeks. The nail plate is the major splint for these injuries and, if intact, they do universally well. Mess up the nail plate and the underlying bone and the likelihood of permanent damage gets higher.

Arthritis

Speaking of permanent damage, with all this wear and tear, the hand may eventually begin to experience the symptoms of arthritis. Those symptoms are pain, swelling and stiffness in a joint. This typically happens in the small joints of the fingers, where it

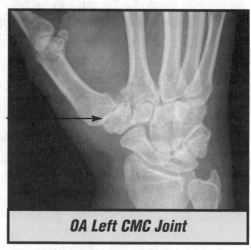

OA Left CMC Joint

commonly begins with the distal joints and heads inward toward the hand. Knobs on that last joint out there by the fingernail are a sign that arthritis is at work. The hand is so busy it may not even notice. These joints are so active that they just have to work, sore or not. They may ache a little in the morning at first, maybe requiring a daily bump of ibuprofen, until finally there are days when that darn finger is getting in the way.

The most common joint of all in which to get significant arthritis is that mobile joint at the base of the thumb. As you've learned, this carpometacarpal ("CMC") joint is a sloppy joint endowed with a great range of motion. It tends to wear out quickest in middle-aged women. In fact, some say this is the most common joint in the body in which women develop osteoarthritis. I'd vote for the knee myself, but the CMC joint is definitely the most common area in the hand. Here it causes pain with grip. The pain is deep at the base of the thumb and, as such, is often either misinterpreted as coming from the adjacent wrist joint or its tendons (e.g. DeQuervain's tendonitis). A physical exam usually localizes the pain to that joint, and sometimes there is a telltale grinding felt in the joint when the thumb is compressed downward along its axis. This "positive grind test"—I'm not kidding; that's what we call it—is another "does-this-hurt?" that we get away with just once in every physical exam. To distinguish this problem from the equally common DeQuervain's syndrome, Dr. Finkelstein's test should be negative. The smart doctor will first do those "provocative maneuvers" he expects to be less painful, saving the best for last. This avoids getting punched in the nose more than once in any single physical examination. If you go straight to the grind test, you may have your diagnosis, but the patient will likely never let you near her thumb again.

Once diagnosed, this condition is usually treated with

reassurance, non-steroidal anti-inflammatory medicines (NSAIDs), sometimes splinting with removable "working splints," or a cortisone shot. It is not unusual for this arthritis to present in fifty-ish women and it can even get to be disabling. When this gets bad, women can't open jars, use shears or scissors, or, in general, do much of anything that involves, thumb pinch. These few unfortunates may need surgery to alleviate the pain. This surgery involves removing the worn out bone at the base of the thumb and putting in some borrowed tendon material as a little cushion. On paper this sounds pretty radical, but in practice it is one of the most tried and true operations in hand surgery. In the past we tried implants of all kinds of things, metal and plastic joint replacements, silastic implants, you name it. They all failed because the stresses are too high and the bones are too small to sustain prostheses. We've been using this "resection arthroplasty" for over 20 years now, and it gives most patients excellent relief.

There is some recent work with newer "pyrolytic carbon" implants that shows promise in replacing some of the small joints of the hand, which previously have not been amenable to joint replacement. I would have to say this work is still at the stage where it is only being done with reliability at major centers doing the research, and is not yet in the "tried and true" category. But

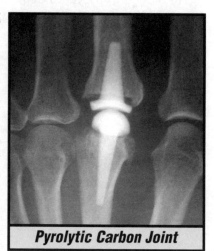

Pyrolytic Carbon Joint

it does show some promise for finger joint replacement in the near future.

So, as you can see, there are a lot of things that can and do go wrong with the boomer hand, so a healthy respect for the vulnerability of the hand is warranted. If you get careless and put your fingers through a band saw, I can tidy it up a bit, but a mangled hand rarely winds up as more than a partly restored, mangled hand. It would better be avoided. Some surgeons are paranoid about their hands, and I think this attitude can be taken to extremes, but I do avoid or eliminate a great many things that put my hands at risk. I can afford not to cut my grass, so I pay someone else to do it. I only use power tools in the operating room and then on you, not me. I avoid un-chaperoned dates with electrical things and sources of power of all kinds. I'm very careful sticking my hands into the dishwater if there are glass or porcelain objects in there. I pay close attention to what I'm doing when I dry a crystal glass. I'm acutely aware that my hands are my livelihood and are constantly at risk. You get the idea. When I get really mad I try to shout something startling as opposed to slugging my yak. People may turn and look at me as if I have Tourette's Syndrome[9], but I won't need an operation or even a cast.

9 Tourette's Syndrome is a bizarre neurological condition in which the sufferer may have explosive verbal tics, such as shouting expletives or even barking.

Chapter 8: The Spine

If you judged orthopedists solely on how we treat problems of the spine, we would get mixed reviews at best. This is a very problematic area for both the patient and the physician, whatever his training. The chances are over 80% that anyone reading this sentence will miss at least some time from work during his lifetime from back pain or neck pain.

Spine Pain is Very Common

- Over 80% of people lose work time with back pain.
- 3 million Americans on disability for back pain
- 3000% increase in disability applications last 20 years
- Third most common reason for surgery in USA
- Second most common reason to visit a doctor
- Fifth most common reason for hospital admission

Spinal pain is almost universal, that is, everybody experiences some sooner or later. If you're lucky it will be short-lived and not disabling. If you're not so lucky, you may have an unwanted friend for life, tagging along on every business trip, showing up like an unwelcome distant relative, moving in and taking over your life for weeks at a time. Many of the maladies of the spine can be attributed to evolution and its affect on a poorly designed skeleton. So, if you don't believe in evolution, I'll guess you just have to blame God outright for lousy workmanship. The main underlying cause of most spinal problems is that we're walking around with a vertical, segmented stack of vertebrae that was originally designed to be a horizontal suspension bridge. If you stood the Golden Gate Bridge up on its Marin County end, it wouldn't work very well either, and that's essentially what's going on with the human spine. Our most distant, segmented-vertebrate ancestors walked on all fours with a horizontal spine. Our nearest ancestors pushed the envelope, transitioning to part-time locomotion on all fours and part-time standing. Only when the Brain saw the distinct advantages of freeing up the hands for more than walking, did we become dominantly bipedal, walkers of the first merit. And that's when the back pain started. I saw a T-shirt on a redneck the other day that said, "I'm not real smart, but I can lift heavy things." I thought, "Yeah, maybe for 15 years, Bubba. Then you're on disability."

The spine is the one area of the orthopedic domain where I no longer wield the knife. I haven't operated on it for about 15 years, so I can't claim any expertise in the surgical management of back conditions. On the other hand, since I specialize in shoulder and hip problems, I frequently see patients with complaints related to the neck and back. Many people who think they have something wrong with their shoulder, in fact, have a neck problem with pains referred to the shoulder. Similarly, back pain is often referred to that area you think of as your "hip." I'll discuss this in more detail later, but trust me, I evaluate a lot of backs and necks. This keeps me familiar with the management of these problems. I also frequently collaborate with both my orthopedic and neurosurgical colleagues.

Bifocal Neck
In the neck we see a host of problems. The deconditioned patient may come in with fatigue presenting as muscular

headache, the fitness nut with pinched nerves from disc degeneration worsened by pounding exercise, the risk-taker may even break his sorry neck rock-climbing or bungee-jumping. But one unique syndrome that is purely a midlife phenomenon is what I call "bifocal neck." This occurs when one's near vision fails, a condition we call "presbyopia," which literally means "aging eyes." You may have been through this process, which begins with the realization that there just isn't enough light to read the menu in the restaurant. Gradually your arms seem too short to extend the page far enough away that you can read it. After a while 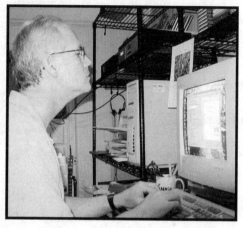 you recognize the problem, which you solve with some of the little reading glasses that sit low on your nose, make you look elderly and are always getting lost. After a year or two you give up and you get some bifocals. For many boomers, this transition happened just as computers were invading the home and the office at an incredible rate. You adapt and the bifocals help. You eventually get pretty adept at cranking your neck up and down to bring the right part of the bifocal into play; thrusting out the chin and pulling the skull back to its legal limit.

This little boogie starts to cause neck pain and sometimes headache, which is muscular in origin, and is especially problematic if you work at a computer. The treatment for this is an awareness of the problem that enables you to orient the subject page or computer screen low enough in your field of vision so that your neck is not strained. Exercises aimed at generalized conditioning of the back and neck, make all these muscular fatigue syndromes easier to tolerate.

Isometric neck-strengthening exercises are simple and can be done at one's desk. First, press both hands against the forehead and hold for a count of five, release and relax, then repeat with the hands behind the head. Complete the cycle pressing the side of the head against the left hand and then the right, in each case holding still for a count of five. Rotate among these four cardinal points, changing hand positions, always pushing against the hand for ten repetitions. If someone says you look funny at your workstation, tell them I told you to do it.

I recently discovered that your eye doctor can make glasses with your bifocal prescription, focused to the exact distance to your computer screen. It's a simple mathematical calculation. I had a pair made and I love them!

Avoiding "Bifocal Neck" Syndrome

- Put computer screen down at bifocal level
- Raise seat relative to screen
- Practice isometric neck exercises
- Prescription computer glasses

Neck Pain and Arthritis

The cervical vertebral discs and the joints between the vertebrae themselves gradually wear with aging. This first starts to show up in the midlife decades. Most neck pain is felt as muscular pain but, in fact, it comes from underlying wear and tear on those two structures that allow the neck its mobility: the cervical discs and the vertebra facet joints.

The human skull is balanced on top of a stack of seven little hatbox shaped vertebrae. Between each is a softer cushion called the intervertebral disc. At the rear of the cervical spine, these vertebra are connected by joints that come together like overlapping tiles on a Spanish roof, two tiles from the vertebra above, overlapping two tiles from the vertebra below. The upper two vertebrae are specialized to provide for more rotation, allowing us to look right

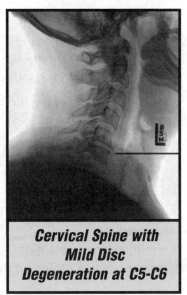

Cervical Spine with Mild Disc Degeneration at C5-C6

and look left for oncoming wildebeests. This stack of vertebrae is supported by a cast of strong muscles, similar to those in the spine that both controls vertebral motion and, in the case of the cervical spine, supports the heavy skull and its special occupant, the Brain. The Brain needs both a sophisticated plumbing system and a very sophisticated wiring system, so these cervical vertebrae double as a structural support tower and a conduit for all the pipes and wires coming and going from the Brain.

So far so good, until the cumulative stresses of forty or fifty years of gravity start to take their toll. The discs wear out and narrow, the little facet joints develop arthritis and the muscles get progressively less able to support the whole system. The resultant condition we call "cervical arthrosis" or "degenerative disc disease." The former is probably the better term in that more than just disc degeneration is involved. This can all be accelerated by injuries major and minor to the discs or to the vertebra themselves.

This cervical arthrosis shows up as pain in the neck and

usually stiffness in the supporting muscles as they go into spasm trying to splint the sore spine. Once again, our current lifestyle is a major contributor to neck pain. Evolution has not had time to adapt to hours spent every day at the computer workstation, or pulling G's in a jet airplane. When I was in the Air Force, I got to take care of a lot of retired fighter pilots. They all had necks that were just scrambled. My wife Kathy and I would joke that we could pick out the former fighter jocks by their C-spine x-rays alone. If your helmet weighs five pounds at one G (normal gravity), it weighs thirty pounds in a six-G turn. Today's F-15 and F-16 fighters can routinely generate nine G's in a split second turn. That causes an enormous stress on the neck and spine.

The patient with cervical arthrosis may experience what he or she interprets as headache and accompanying neck pain and stiffness. The physical exam is usually non-specific, but may show some limitation of spinal motion, muscle spasm and perhaps even some noise (creaking) with motion. The doc will always do a rather sophisticated neurological examination, looking specifically for signs of nerve or spinal cord involvement, but this will rarely yield any clues. The x-ray will show some worn out discs and arthritis in the facet joints.

At this stage, the doctor is often bored because he has nothing fancy to offer. There is no surgery for this condition. Patients honestly don't want a lecture on vertebral evolution, no matter how erudite it may be. They want something to get rid of their pain and stiffness. We can offer NSAIDs, and recommend exercises directed at strengthening the muscles that support the neck. These actually help, but patients rarely do them consistently. If one isolated disc can be identified as the main source of pain, sometimes fusing that segment surgically will temporarily alleviate the "pain generator." But there's a price to pay. Down the line, a fused segment places more stress on the adjacent vertebral segments, causing the next disc down the line to give out. There is a recurring theme here: *operating on spinal pain alone is rarely effective. Whereas, operating on pinched nerves from some spinal cause is often helpful.* You will hear me say this throughout the chapter. Many physical modalities such as heat, massage, stretching and brief immobilization in a soft collar may help cervical arthrosis, but, in general, this is a chronic condition for which there is only palliative therapy.

So, cervical arthrosis is not a condition with a very sunny outlook. But paying attention to a number of lifestyle factors can help somewhat. Boomers who suffer neck pain in the work place should carefully consider modifying their job description to avoid prolonged gazing at the computer screen. Modifying your sleeping habits, particularly through something as mundane as pillow selection, may help this problem too. I have a C6-C7 disc degeneration and can only sleep on a very firm, rather high foam pillow. For me it's enough of an issue that I am willing to lug a "travel pillow" version of my home pillow with me whenever I'm on the road. I've found that this makes all the difference in the world.

What Works for Neck Arthritis

Good things are:
- Cervical isometric exercises
- Home traction
- NSAIDs
- Pillow modifications/neck pillows
- Generalized aerobic conditioning

Cervical Radiculopathy

If your doctor seemed bored after examining your neck for that pain you've been having, it was because he hoped he might find the signs of a pinched nerve and didn't. While cervical arthrosis only calls into sharp focus our inadequacy as healers, a pinched nerve is something for which we can help you.

A pinched nerve in the neck is called a "cervical radiculopathy." The nerve roots that exit the spinal cord pass out between adjacent vertebra and right beside the discs, Since these nerves are on their way to the arm and hand, anything that pinches the nerve in the neck will usually be felt in the shoulder, arm, forearm or hand. As is the case with any pinched nerve, the symptoms can be any combination of pain, sensory change (numbness, burning etc), or weakness in the muscles supplied by that particular nerve.

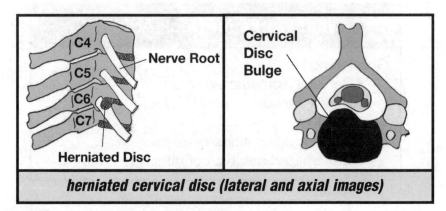

herniated cervical disc (lateral and axial images)

There are five main nerve roots that exit from the cervical spine and pass from the neck down to the upper extremity. Pinching any specific one of these produces a completely different distribution of symptoms. The beauty of a well-conducted physical examination for this condition is that it can zero in on the exact problem, incriminating a specific nerve or nerves. The most common disc herniations and nerve root compressions occur at the C5-C6 disc, causing a cervical radiculopathy that involves the C6 nerve root. So let's take that as an example.

A patient comes to my office with a chief complaint of shoulder and arm pain. An avid jogger, he relates a history of pain in his right arm that he first noticed after running. The pain began in the muscles along the right side of his neck, and then spread over the shoulder and down the lateral side of his arm. He assumed it was a shoulder problem, but for some reason it didn't really hurt when he moved his shoulder. In fact, it was often worse at night, when he lay down to sleep. Gradually, he noticed that he was having more trouble flexing his elbow. It just felt weaker when he was lifting heavy things, such as the two-year old from his second marriage to the trophy wife—but that's another story. Over the last week he has noticed a burning pain that goes all the way down to his thumb. It's not there all the time but comes and goes rather suddenly. When I ask him if there's anything that aggravates these symptoms, he offers that sneezing is so painful that he has come to dread it. When I ask if anything relieves the pain, he says, "Funny you should mention it, but I can make the pain a lot better by putting my hand on the top of my head."

BINGO! Only a cervical radiculopathy will do that. In fact, this little clue (which is infrequent) is so specific that we call it "pathognomonic" of a pinched nerve in the neck, meaning that this specific symptom is seen only with a cervical radiculopathy. I examine the patient, and I discover that he has some pain with neck motion, particularly when I move his head toward the sore shoulder. However, he has no real pain when I put the shoulder through its paces. He does have a weak biceps muscle and, more importantly, when I tap the biceps tendon to provoke the little reflex that normally should be there, it isn't. He also has slightly decreased sensation when tested with a pin along the back of his thumb. The x-rays show mild narrowing of the C5-C6 disc, but not much else. I order an MRI of his neck and it confirms a herniation of the disc at that level, pinching on the sixth cervical nerve root. Because of the weakness and reflex changes, I refer him immediately to either an orthopedic spine surgeon or a neurosurgeon. Here again, "all politics is local." In some areas orthopedists are the ones who handle this problem, and in others it's the neurosurgeons. In many other locales, doctors duke it out for these patients.

In mild cases without significant neurological deficits, such as weakness or reflex changes, we usually start with just cervical traction. We send the patients to the physical therapist and they hook them up with a system of pulleys, a head halter and weights. They sit under this traction apparatus getting their neck stretched for a while. There are also fancier units that have the patient lie down and use his body as counter traction. This may be combined with a cervical collar. As long as there is no progressive nerve deficit, and the patient shows some signs of improvement, traction alone may be an effective therapy. If not, surgery is indicated.

Sometimes, the diagnosis is not so easy to make. The patient may have a mixed picture of cervical radiculopathy *and* shoulder problems such as rotator cuff tendonitis. In these cases, we may send the patient to the "interventional" radiologist for a selective nerve block. These guys will skillfully put a needle near the nerve root at just the level in question and inject it with anesthetic and sometimes cortisone. If this relieves the pain, it helps us to make the diagnosis of cervical radiculopathy.

The surgery for this condition involves removing whatever is pinching on the nerve root. Usually, this is a herniated disc, but spurs from the adjacent vertebral joints may also be contributing to the problem. This surgery is called "cervical discectomy" and is most commonly done through an incision on the front of the neck that carefully moves through all the pipes and wires that keep the brain comfortably plumbed and connected. This is sophisticated surgery to say the least and should only be done by surgeons specifically trained in these techniques. In many cases the failed disc is fused by placing a bone graft in the disc space, preserving the height of the vertebral column and preventing further disc herniation or narrowing.

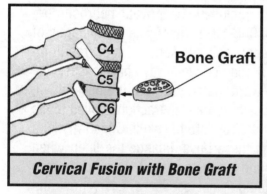

Cervical Fusion with Bone Graft

Treatment of Pinched Nerve in the Neck

- Cervical traction
- Cervical nerve root injections
- NSAIDs
- Rest and time
- If pain not resolving or if progressive nerve impairment, then surgery to remove herniated disc, possible fusion

C-spine Fractures and Paralysis

There are some subjects in medicine that just give us doctors the creeps, and for me this is one of them. Nothing is so gut-wrenching or tragic as seeing a young person who, moments before his injury, was not only walking but often pursuing some joyous physical activity like diving into a lake or playing football. Here I know more sad stories than I want to think about. I probably need go no further than to remind you of Christopher Reeves, but I have some personal examples that haunt my dreams. Quadraplegia and kidney failure are probably my greatest fears. They are the monsters that live under my bed.

While I was an undergraduate, I worked as an orderly and nurses' aide at the University Hospitals in Iowa City. This is how I paid my way through my pre-medical years in college. The ward I worked on included the private neurosurgery patients. At this time, 1968-1971, there was an epidemic of football related cervical spine fractures and resulting permanent paralyses. It seemed we always had at least one teenage athlete on the ward, paralyzed from the neck down, lying on a special sandwich frame with traction applied to his head through tongs sunk deep into the skull. One of my jobs was to wash and bathe these guys, change the linen when their sphincters failed, and flip them in their sandwich frames every hour so they wouldn't get bedsores. Every now and then the tongs placed in someone's skull would pull out of the bone and a loud "clank" would echo down the hall as the twenty or twenty-five pounds of traction weights crashed to the floor. Helpless, the patient would cry out, unable to so much as push the nurse's call button. Though these guys were exactly my age, there I was, alive and well, my whole life in medicine before me. There they were, helpless, at the mercy of others, their whole paralyzed lives before them. It just tore my heart out.

At the level of the cervical spine where most fractures and dislocations of the vertebra occur, there is little tolerance for displacement. Even the slightest fracture will almost certainly injure this vulnerable tissue, and the resultant paralysis is profound and permanent. You do see the occasional football player who suffers a "temporary" paralysis, but these usually involve what is essentially a contusion or bruise of the spinal cord and usually are not associated with a significant fracture or dislocation. When the spine is bent too far in the wrong direction, or loaded suddenly end-on, as when a player "spears" another player he is tackling with his helmet, the spine either fractures, is dislocated, or both. Either calamity is curtains for the spinal cord.

Some athletes are actually predisposed to spinal cord injury and may not know it. They may be discovered to have a congenitally narrow spine, only after a frightening episode of transient paralysis. Here's where seeing yourself in one of my "Boomer Syndromes" gets serious. If you're a risk taker you should think very seriously about paralysis as a possible consequence of your actions. Sure, you can get pithed driving to work; that happens sometimes. But skiing into a tree or falling from a hang-glider or coming up a little long on a bungee jump sure is something you can avoid. With the epidemic of "Boomeritis," it seems to me that becoming paralyzed for life is one of those calamities that is just way too scary to risk. With so many ways to be entertained and so many ways to stay fit, why someone would select an activity that consistently puts the spinal cord at risk is beyond me.

Yes, the treatments we have nowadays to stabilize the fractured spine are better than those we had when I was caring for these kids back in the 1960s. And yes, there have been some advances in the rehabilitation of these injuries, surgical and otherwise. But do you really want to be stabilized and rehabilitated? As Arlo Guthrie said in *Alice's Restaurant,* "Son, have you rehabilitated yourself?"

The Thoracic Spine

That part of the spine where the ribs attach is called the "thoracic spine." Of all the three mobile regions of the spine, this one is the least affected by arthritis, disc degeneration and nerve compression. Or perhaps it would be more accurate to say that since there is less relative motion among these thoracic segments and their job is primarily to work with the ribs in protecting the vital chest organs (the heart, lungs and major vessels), the thoracic spine suffers less wear and tear.

Although sometimes we see the rare herniated thoracic disc, the two most common conditions we treat are pain from poor posture and, in some women in midlife, early osteoporosis.

Osteoporosis is a complicated subject. For a more complete discussion of its causes, diagnosis and treatment, I suggest you read *Chapter 13: Osteoporosis.* Here I'll simply say that many forty and fifty year-old women may have already begun to suffer from the early signs of this condition, which include softening of the vertebral bodies and a gradual exaggerated rounding of the thoracic curvature. These problems place excessive strain on the muscles of the spine in this region, which support the head and anchor the shoulders to the thorax. Women (and some men) who have this condition can feel a build up of tension right between the shoulder blades. The two keys to treatment here are actually prevention of osteoporosis with calcium supplementation and simple conditioning exercises to strengthen the muscles that extend the spine. Strengthening these muscles make them more resistant to fatigue.

Prevention of Kyphosis

- Extension exercises
- Calcium supplementation
- In some cases estrogen and/or bisphosphonates (Fosamax)

...in other words, prevention of osteoporosis and its fractures

---

The Lower Back

Of all the orthopedic problems we see, the lower back is probably the greatest source of lost workdays, disability, misery and remorse. It is estimated that 80% of working Americans will be forced to take some time off from work due to backache. Here the cumulative effects of obesity, gravity, and entropy come home to roost just above the belt. We call the lower back the "lumbar spine." Essentially, we're talking about the last five vertebra and their discs, the little cushions between them that allow segmental motion. I guess I should really say, the last five vertebrae that move and have discs. In animals with tails, there are more segments below what we call the lumbar spine. In humans, however, these motion segments have fused

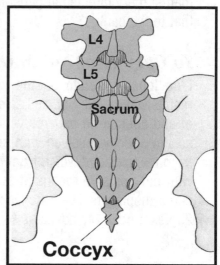

into one bone, the sacrum, that immobile part of the spine that is the central keystone of the pelvis.

Herein lies the problem. Anywhere in the skeleton where something that moves meets something that doesn't move, there is a concentration of stress. Any architect would

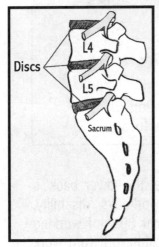

look at the spine and predict that the weakest link would be where the mobile, segmented lumbar spine meets the immobile, rigid sacrum. And it is here that over 90% of disc problems and most of the degenerative conditions congregate.

In the simplest rendering, low back problems fit into two categories: localized back pain, and pain at some distance (usually in the leg) caused by pinched nerves that exit the spine at the lumbar level. Surgery is most helpful for the latter and least helpful for the former. In other words, surgery to relieve pinched nerve pain is more likely to result in a happy patient than surgery directed at general low back pain. You can take that to the bank.

To Operate or Not to Operate

I no longer operate on the spine and never enjoyed the results when I did. But, as I said above, I frequently take care of and operate on patients with shoulder pain and hip pain, so I'm directly involved with sorting out which pain comes from the neck and which from the back. Since I work closely with our spinal surgeons at the clinic, both neurosurgeons and orthopedists, I've watched the results of surgery for over 25 years now. My advice is to be very wary of the surgeon who promises, or even suggests, that he or she can remedy your low back pain with an operation. Only consent to surgery that is directed at relieving pain going down into the leg, and only when a reasonable period of conservative management has been tried.

Most surgeons who operate on the back would agree that the indications for spinal surgery are confined to those pinched nerves that result in some neurological deficit, such as weakness in the leg muscles or disturbance of bowel or bladder function; unremitting pain from a pinched nerve; a few spinal deformities like scoliosis (and even then the result is more cosmetic than pain controlling); and, of course, various fractures and tumors. Operating on just back pain usually results in more back pain and a scar. In fact, we doctors don't know exactly what causes most back pain. That may sound outrageous, but it's true. Simplistic concepts that link back pain to spinal instability, disc degeneration, arthritis of the joints between the vertebrae or muscular spasm are at best incomplete. Most back pain probably involves a complex interplay of several causes and, therefore, is not amenable to some simple surgical solution.

An excellent recent article in the August 8th, 2002 edition of *The New Yorker* by Dr. Jerome Groopman[10], titled "Knife in the Back" described this problem in layman's terms and I recommend it highly. His basic point is that not only is the cause of back pain incompletely understood, but the treatment you receive is essentially a "franchise" of the type of doctor you see. Surgeons think mechanically and prescribe surgical solutions; rheumatologists think medically and prescribe medicines; physical medicine doctors (physiatrists) prescribe therapy; radiologists stick needles in things etc. But in the end, since we don't honestly know what we're treating, the best treatments are those that do the

10 http://www.jeromegroopman.com/knife.html

least harm.

So that's the bad news. The good news is that nowhere is the old saw "an ounce of prevention is worth a pound of cure" more true than in the back. Most of the patients we see with chronic low back problems are deconditioned, sedentary and overweight; have weak abdominal and trunk muscles; and smoke. Yes, even smoking contributes to low back pain by somehow contributing to disc degeneration. You can decrease your risk for serious back problems by avoiding nicotine, losing weight, strengthening the trunk muscles, increasing your aerobic fitness and avoiding repetitive impact loading activities, such as jogging, long distance driving and step-aerobics. The highest stress loads on the discs are caused by flexion and rotation, so be careful about bending over and twisting at the same time. A good example of a high-risk situation would be that little bit of hand-to-hand combat that goes on at the baggage carousel where you're leaning over between two other boomers, twisting to get at that overstuffed bag. It's worth the tip to let the Sky Cap do that work. You can also focus on strengthening those abdominal muscles that support the back from the front of the body. Because of its mechanically disadvantaged position behind the body's center of gravity, the lumbar spine is very dependent on the muscular support of the belly muscles. When properly conditioned, these muscles pull the spine into flexion to balance the spinal muscles that extend it. Many of the patients I see in the clinic with backache cannot even sit up on the exam table without the help of their arms to push them up.

Decreasing the Risk for Back Pain

- Don't smoke!
- Stay near ideal weight
- Practice aerobic conditioning
- Avoid heavy lifting
- Strengthen trunk muscles
- Avoid impact loading sports (jogging, jumping)

On the treatment side, once you have a backache, there are few things that have been shown to help more than the tincture of time. There is some evidence for the following: rest but not bed-rest, analgesics but not narcotics, spinal manipulation in cases without pinched nerves, exercise and massage. There is little or no evidence for the use of corsets, traction, bed-rest, injections, and the host of other poultices and potions. Despite the lack of scientific evidence to support their use—-and perhaps because of this lack—-there has erupted a whole industry of whimsical "alternative" treatments for low back pain. You've seen the anti-gravity boots and the various vibrators, massagers, etc. This is a multi-million dollar industry, which is an outgrowth of our inability to offer anything more than "take two aspirin and call me in the morning." And we prefer a morning about six weeks from now.

Things That Work for Back Pain

- Rest but not recumbence
- NSAIDs but not narcotics or muscle relaxants
- Exercise but not traction
- Massage and maybe manipulation
- Bracing but only temporarily
- Time

When it comes to surgery, even for herniated discs that press on the spinal nerves (sciatica), there is only scant evidence that patients are better off one year after surgery than they would have been without surgery. It is clear that for sciatica from a herniated disc, patients do get better quicker with surgery and therefore it is justified. But again, the only firm surgical indications are for evolving or progressing neurological deficits. This means a muscle that has been weakened because the nerve supplying it is pinched, or perhaps numbness that is progressing. Remember that the nerves that exit the back carry the nerve impulses to the muscles, and carry sensation from the surface of the limb back to the spinal cord and the brain. If the nerve pinched at the level of the disc is causing progressive muscle weakness or numbness, this suggests that more permanent nerve damage is imminent. Most surgeons agree that this situation justifies operating on the spine. Yet, when you follow those who have had surgery for long enough, the evidence is not convincing that performing surgery makes people any better than if you had simply waited. However, surgery certainly does get patients quicker pain relief in these specific cases.

Bottom line: think twice about any back surgery, and then think a third time. Some of the most miserable patients we see are those "failed backs" who have had two, three or four unsuccessful surgical attempts to cut out the pain. Luckily, most spine surgeons are just as conservative as their patients should be and will advise against all but the most clearly indicated operations. They want to have good results too.

For these reasons, as I discuss the most common conditions that affect the lower back—herniated discs, degenerative disc disease and its sequelae (which include spinal stenosis), and a few less common conditions that may afflict the boomer spine—I will emphasize a conservative, preventive approach, heavily weighted toward exercise, physical therapy, and maintenance. My motto is: "Ask not what your doctor can do for your back; ask what *you* can do for *your own* back, and then do it!"

"Slipped" Discs

You hear this all the time, "Bonnie slipped a disc and had to have it removed." In order to understand what is really going on here, we have to review the anatomy of the lumbar spine. I touched on this above, but here the relationship between the vertebrae (the bones), the discs (the cartilage cushions between the bones) and the spinal nerves that exit the spine, is critical to understanding what goes wrong. Let's look at that diagram again. Focus on the

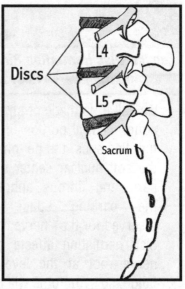

last two vertebrae, which we call the fourth and fifth lumbar vertebrae (L4 and L5). The disc between them is labeled the L4-5 disc. Between each two vertebrae a spinal nerve exits through the gap made by the vertebra above and the vertebra below, in this case L4 above and L5 below. This happens on each side, so there is a nerve root going left and a nerve root going to the right.

As they exit, these spinal nerve roots pass near the disc. If the disc is doing its job, is healthy and standing tall, there is plenty of room for the nerves to exit. But if the disc is worn out, it may bulge outward and collapse vertically, restricting the space available for the spinal nerve root. We call this

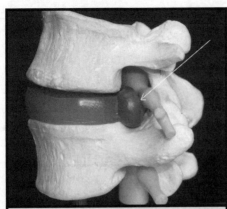

Lumbar Disc Herniation Pinching Exiting Nerve Root

outward bulging of the disc a "herniation," and it is this disc herniation that has morphed into the slang, "slipped disc."

Looking even closer, we can see that the disc is not a homogenous structure but more like a candy with a softer center. The edge of the disc (the "annulus," as we call it) is made of strong fibrous tissue that restrains the softer, central portion of the disc we call the "nucleus." As the disc ages, the peripheral fibers wear out and may allow the soft nuclear center to escape, or herniate, through the peripheral fibrous annulus into the parking space usually reserved for the nerve root. This disc herniation affects only the nerve root at the level of the bulge, so symptoms will be felt in the leg, but only where that nerve root is going. This is one thing that makes pinched nerve pain so variable and mysterious. If you know the anatomy of where these nerves go, the patient's symptoms make sense. But even experienced physicians may mistake the pain from a pinched lumbar nerve root for a hip, knee, leg or foot problem. Nerves that exit the lumbar spine supply all these areas and a herniated disc

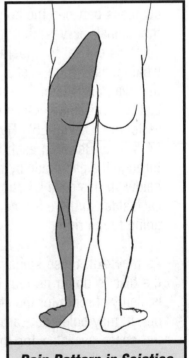

Pain Pattern in Sciatica

176

can cause pain in any of these regions. This whole syndrome of leg pain from a pinched nerve is often called "sciatica," referring to irritation of the sciatic nerve at one of its contributing nerve roots. I tell my patients to imagine the sciatic nerve as an upside down tree with the roots in your back, the trunk coming out of your pelvis in your butt and the branches going down your leg. If you pinch one of the roots, the branches supplied by that root will be symptomatic, just as when you cut one root to a tree. The whole tree doesn't die, but the branches supplied by that root will suffer.

After the initial event—the disc herniation—there is a period of inflammation and swelling around the squashed nerve root. This is the period during which the nerve pain is at its worst. It may completely immobilize the patient with both back pain and leg pain, almost always on just one side since the herniation is usually forced to one side, affecting either the right or left nerve root at that level. In these cases we recommend rest; strong, usually narcotic painkillers; drugs to lessen the inflammation and sometimes drugs to control muscle spasm. While rest and anti-inflammatories may lessen the reaction around the nerve root, and the pain medicines certainly help by dulling the pain, most of the so-called "muscle-relaxants" probably work only as chemical restraints—they dope the patient up so much that he has no alternative but to stay in bed. These drugs are also notoriously addicting and few spine surgeons actually prescribe them anymore.

The patient with an acute disc herniation should be examined for signs of muscle weakness, loss of sensation (numbness), loss of certain reflexes ("So that's why he hit me with that little hammer!"), and, in the worst cases, bowel or bladder disturbance. These are more serious signs. If they are present in the beginning and not improving quickly, the surgeon will usually recommend surgery to relieve pressure on the nerve. An alternative that is employed more frequently these days is a type of cortisone injection around the nerve root where it is pinched. This is called a "lumbar epidural steroid injection." *Lumbar* describes the location in the spine; *epidural* means around but not into the nerve root, *steroid* is an alias for cortisone; and if you don't know what an injection is, I give up.

What Makes You Think You Have a Herniated Lumbar Disc?

- Pain is often "electrical" and worse down the leg than in the back
- Pain may be migratory–moving from one area of the buttock or leg to another
- Any combination of pain, numbness and weakness
- Leg pain may have been foreshadowed by back pain

Somewhere during the diagnostic process, doctors have to gather a little more information to be sure of what we're treating and where to use either the needle or the knife. In the old days, this meant an invasive test called a myelogram in which the doctor did a spinal tap and then filled the sac around the spinal nerves with a dye that showed up on x-ray. Then the patient was rolled around on the x-ray table and tilted every which way to get the dye to fill the area around the nerve roots. A herniated disc showed up on the myelogram as an indentation in the dye or a deviation of the nerve root away from its expected path. This was indirect, circumstantial evidence at best. Today the testing has become both non-invasive (most of the time we don't stick you with anything) and much more reliable. Today's MRI[11]

11 MRI stands for "magnetic resonance imaging."

tests of the spine are a truly remarkable advance, and show the disc, the nerve root, the bones, the ligaments, and sometimes, even tumors and other unexpected things we might never have found otherwise. Anybody with a herniated disc who is not improving with conservative management should have an MRI of the spine.

As with any test, there are limitations. Here the problem is that the "M" in MRI stands for "magnetic." If you have any strategically placed metal objects in your body—oh say, a clip on a blood vessel in your brain, or a pacemaker tick-tocking your heart—you're out of luck. It's considered poor form to have the patient's brain slam up against the MRI machine or for his pacemaker to go flying out of his chest like

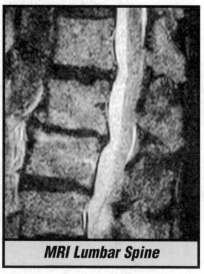

MRI Lumbar Spine

something from the movie, *Alien*. Contrary to popular myth, a lot of the hardware we orthopods leave lying around inside of patients is either not ferromagnetic or, if it is, it is not at great risk of coming unglued. In cases where an MRI is not an option, the spine can still be imaged with sophisticated CAT scans, sometimes combined with the older technique of myelography. Once the spine is imaged, the questions become: 1) At what disc level is the herniation and how big is it? 2) What nerve root(s) is/are affected and how badly? 3) Should we operate and, if so, what technique should we use? The MRI or CAT scan can answer numbers one and two. The surgeon and the patient have to decide together on number three.

Good Reasons to Have Surgery for Herniated Lumbar Disc

- Persistent sciatica (lower extremity pain) despite conservative treatment
- Progressive weakness, numbness or pain
- Good but temporary response to nerve root or epidural injection
- Pain pattern, neurological exam and imaging (MRI etc.) all fit

Currently there are several accepted techniques for removing a herniated disc but they all boil down to making an opening in the back down to the spine, removing only enough bone to get into the area of the nerve root and the disc (a laminectomy), retracting the nerve root out of harm's way, and cutting out the herniated portion of the disc and any other disc material that might become herniated later (discectomy). How big to make the incision, what specific tools to use, whether to fuse the disc or use a microscope to assist in the procedure—-all these decisions are variable. But all techniques share laminectomy and discectomy through some sort of incision. If you're not bored by now, I am, so let's make this a little more human with a patient example.

Every now and then someone decides that the morbidity of laminectomy is just too much and there's got to be an easier way. In the early 1980s someone decided that it would be easier to just inject something that digested the disc itself. No incision; no scar; less pain; quicker recovery; just put a needle in the disc and eat it up. It was determined that this could be done with an enzyme derived from the papaya plant. I'm not making this up, folks. I'm dead serious. This chemical was called "chymopapain," and these types of injections were all the rage in the early 1980s when I was in private practice in Iowa. And I'll admit it did seem attractive. Rather than cut through the spinal muscles and the bone, retract the nerve root and physically cut out the herniated disc, this procedure offered the chance of just injecting this papaya stuff into the disc under local anesthetic. In goes the chymopapain; out goes the pain.

I went to a course in Chicago, sponsored at least in part by the company who made this drug. There I learned the techniques of needle placement, how to inject dye into the disc in order to be sure the needle was where it was supposed to be and so forth.

After I came back from the course, I still wasn't sold. In fact, I had not yet injected any patients with chymopapain when one day a little flyer from the drug company came in the mail. It said there had been 18 or so cases of "acute transverse myelitis" associated with chymopapain injection. All had been connected to injections of dye into the disc (the very technique they had been recommending at this course) and now they no longer recommended injecting dye, just the papaya juice. I thought, "Acute transverse myelitis? Doesn't that mean IMMEDIATE, IRREVERSBLE PARALYSIS FROM THE WAIST DOWN?" What they were saying was that their drug had caused at least 18 cases of patients permanently paralyzed from a procedure meant to be a "less invasive" alternative than simple discectomy. Many lawsuits did arise, and chymopapain injections rapidly fell out of favor. For this reason and others, I began to sour on back surgery in general, but that's not part of this story.

In the intervening 20 years, doctors have flirted with a number of other techniques for disc eradication on behalf of treating back pain. The current one involves placing a curved needle that can conduct heat through a high radio-frequency into the disc. This is supposed to melt and shrink the disc (I guess), thus avoiding open discectomy. My advice to anyone thinking about letting his doctor try a new technique on him is to first let someone play around with it for about five years. Wait until a large number of cases with a high success rate and a correspondingly low complication rate have been published before you sign up for this or any other new procedure. Standard, open laminectomy and discectomy, usually with the assistance of the microscope, is the gold standard surgical procedure for a diagnosed herniated disc that has not responded to non-surgical management. And remember: this is a treatment directed at alleviating the leg pain, not at the back pain.

Accepted Surgical Alternatives for Herniated Lumbar Disc

- Traditional "open" laminectomy
- Micro-laminectomy
- In cases with instability, laminectomy and fusion

Degenerative Disc Disease

The isolated, herniated disc is actually a rare event compared to the common wear and tear we call "degenerative disc disease." In any other joint system, we call this arthritis. I say joint "system" because the spine works together as a series of stacked joints, each with one vertebra above and one below joined by the

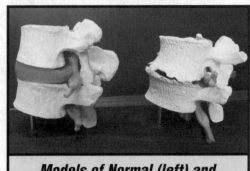

Models of Normal (left) and Degenerated Lumbar Disc (right)

disc and by true synovial joints behind, which we call the facet joints. We've visited this territory before, but now let's look at what happens when the system just wears out.

As the disc ages, it dries out and gets less effective at resisting the compressive forces it is designed to cushion. In other words, it becomes a less efficient shock absorber. This eventually leads to more stress on the facet joints behind. They undergo the same type of degenerative arthritis that we see in the knee or hip, complete with the loss of joint cartilage and the development of those bone spurs we call osteophytes. Just as with degenerative arthritis anywhere, the person experiences associated pain, stiffness and usually muscle spasm as the back tries to splint its damaged joints. The ensuing pain may be acute, chronic or a little of both, with a baseline ache that is there all the time, interspersed with sudden episodes of excruciating, sometimes incapacitating, take-your-breath-away pain.

What Makes You Think You Have Lumbar Degenerative Disc Disease?

- Chronic, midline low back pain with ups and downs
- Pain is often at the beltline or just above
- Pain may radiate into buttocks
- Pain often associated with muscle spasm
- Often runs a painful ten-year course, then burns out

An x-ray at this time will be rather non-specific, showing some worn out discs, some spurs, narrowed facet joints and the overall picture that we label "degenerative disc disease." The tough thing is that, unlike arthritis elsewhere, there is really no surgical remedy for this problem. We can offer all the usual supportive modalities—rest, heat, pain medicines, physical therapy etc.—but they have little effect on the underlying condition and are at best palliative. The patient and, of course, the surgeon would like some quick, effective, often surgical treatment to be rid of this pain, but, alas, there is none. Yet, so often that doesn't keep the well-intentioned surgeon from offering the patient what sounds like a logical surgical "correction" for the problem. The surgeon may offer a fusion—an operation designed to take away the pain by taking away the motion at the specific vertebral segment that is supposed to be causing the pain. If he does an MRI, the degenerated disc will show up dark and sinister, what is often called a "black disc." Since this looks so ominous, it is easy to understand the seduction of this simple plan: find the disc that's causing the problem; fuse it and the problem will go away. The only problem is that there is precious little evidence that this procedure works, and abundant evidence that fusion is not a predictable treatment for back pain from degenerative disc disease.

The Golden Rule of Spine Surgery

"The best results are when you are operating on the spine to relieve pinched nerve pain. In the low back that means leg pain and in the neck that means arm pain."

We are back to the axioms I proposed in the opening part of this chapter. Surgery is usually not effective when directed at back pain alone. Spine surgery is most effective for leg pain from a herniated disc, for certain fractures, and for a few spinal deformities and pinched nerves from spinal arthritis, a condition I'll discuss in the next section. But for degenerative disc disease alone, that is causing primarily low back pain, the treatment is rest for the acute episodes, trunk-strengthening exercises done *forever*, weight control, NSAIDs, and generalized conditioning. This is extremely hard to get across to the patient with an acutely painful back. But if he could only see a few of those "failed backs" who have had five or six operations, whose x-rays are encrusted with hardware and who are much worse off than when they first consented to surgery, he'd be a believer. Failed backs are among the most miserable people on the planet. The most common patients seen in "chronic pain management" centers, they are typically addicted to narcotics and chronically disabled. Their lives are disasters and they are paying the price of a society that worships technology above reason.

Here are some more sobering statistics. At any given point in time, six million Americans are on disability for back pain. Around 3 million are now on permanent disability for low back pain. Since 1980 there has been a 3000% increase in applications for disability for back pain. Back pain (not herniated disc, just back pain) is the third most common reason for surgery in the United States. It is the second most common reason for a patient visiting the doctor and the fifth most common reason for admission to the hospital. These statistics are completely unique to the United States and are not seen in any other industrialized country. The reason? We consider back pain to have a compensable cause, to have a surgical treatment and to be a reason not to work. More is spent per year on the treatment of back pain than on NASA or the Human Genome Project. And remember this is all spent on treatment of a condition for which we do not actually understand the cause. It's staggering, but one estimate of the direct and indirect cost of back pain is over thirty billion dollars per year in this country.

So, obviously, my advice to you, fellow boomer, is to avoid the knife. It is rarely the treatment for back pain. Do the exercises, take the medicines, avoid the narcotics, and wait it out. Though it may never go away, it will likely get better and probably much better than if you have something fused.

Spinal Stenosis

"Stenosis" means a narrowing or constriction. In the lumbar spine, spinal stenosis refers to the narrowing of the spinal canal that results from chronic degenerative disc disease. As the discs age and wear out, they lose their height, narrowing the space available for the exiting spinal nerves by collapsing the space between the vertebrae. The spurs that arise from the arthritic facet joints further narrow the spinal canal, pinching on the spinal nerves, often on both sides and at several vertebral levels.

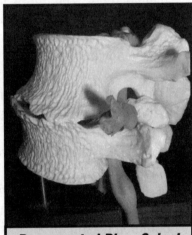

Degenerated Disc, Spinal Stenosis, Narrowing of Nerve Outlet

What the patient experiences is numbness and weakness in the legs. These neurological symptoms are usually related to walking and to certain activities, such as walking downhill or standing for a while. Like other pinched nerve symptoms— sciatica from a herniated disc, for instance—spinal stenosis can be relieved by surgery. Here we are revisiting a theme: back surgery works for pinched nerve or leg symptoms but not for back pain alone.

Spinal stenosis is a relatively simple diagnosis to make. The patient usually complains of a long history of gradually increasing symptoms of leg numbness, a dead or heavy feeling in the legs with exertion or, sometimes, pain in the buttocks and legs when walking or standing. These symptoms have to be separated from the other possible causes of leg pain from walking, especially circulatory causes. We call cramping and pain with walking "claudication," and we usually think of vascular claudication in older people who have hardening of the arteries from smoking, diabetes or high cholesterol. The symptoms of spinal stenosis are so similar that they are sometimes called "neurogenic claudication," implying that the underlying cause is a pinching of the nerves in the lumbar spine and not poor circulation. The reason the diagnosis is usually easy is because the patient with vascular claudication usually has other signs of poor circulation and often doesn't have palpable pulses in the feet. The diagnosis can be clinched by the combination of a good history, a physical exam focused on sorting out poor pulses, the usual findings on the back x-ray, an MRI showing the spinal canal narrowing and sometimes blood pressure tests of the circulation.

The surgery for spinal stenosis involves freeing up the pinched nerves by cleaning out the spurs, the thickened ligaments and anything else pinching on them. This surgery is extensive but usually successful. It may involve taking away enough bone that the vertebrae need to be stabilized with a fusion at one or more levels. This may require spinal hardware such as screws and rods and possibly bone grafting to achieve solid fusion. But the important thing is the decompression of the nerves as they exit the spine. If this can be done without rendering the spine unstable, the surgeon will avoid hardware. We're talking about cutting out the facet joints and the discs that hold the vertebrae together. If so much bone must be resected that it renders the spine

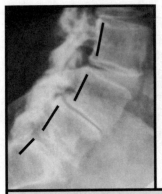

sloppy, or might allow one vertebra to slide forward on another, then instrumentation will be used to hold the fusion.

Spinal stenosis surgery is in the same category as surgery for a herniated disc. It involves operating on the spine to relieve symptoms in the legs. Though it is clearly major

Decompressed Lumbar Spine with Some Instability, Forward Slippage of Vertebra

surgery and not to be taken lightly, it is predictably effective—at relieving the nerve symptoms, though not always the back pain.

Spondylolysis

There is a common spinal defect that sometimes doesn't really show up until the boomer years. "Spondylo" means spine and "lysis" means dissolution or loosening. Together they refer to a specific defect that occurs in the lowest lumbar vertebra, usually at L5. This defect is usually not present at birth and is actually thought to be a fatigue or stress fracture. We encounter these also in the hip, foot and tibia. These fractures occur when the bone is stressed beyond its limit through cycle after cycle of loading, as seen in the so-called "march facture" of the foot bones in military recruits. This particular stress fracture occurs in the critical area at the back of the last vertebra, probably from the high concentration of loading stresses

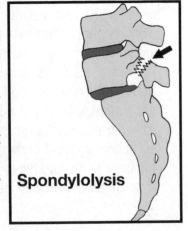

Spondylolysis

there. A defect here not only causes localized pain, but sometimes allows the whole spinal column above to slide forward, a condition we call "spondylolisthesis," where "spondylo" is once again a Latin alias for spine and "listhesis" is a ten-dollar doctor's word for slippage. Thus you can have the poetical combination of spondylolysis *and* spondylolisthesis.

Spondylolysis is often the result of some of the Syndromes I discussed earlier. It is very common in jumping sports, gymnastics and weightlifting. My brother the state-champion high jumper had this. One of my friend's wives who was a high-performance gymnast had this. Remember that famous picture of Olga Korbut in the 1972 Munich Olympics, arched back on the balance beam with her butt over her head? That's the sort of thing that leads to spondylolysis. There is a fairly high prevalence of this condition among NFL linemen, again, presumably from lifting so much heavy weight to build muscle and strength.

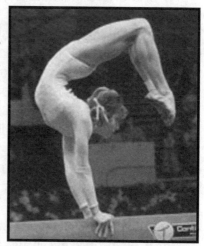

The boomer with this condition shows up in the clinic with midline, beltline low back pain. The more advanced cases may experience some irritation of the L5 nerve root because it passes out at this level, but most patients have a combination of pain and muscle spasm. Like all other types of back pain, the initial treatment for this problem is conservative and not surgical. But this is one exception to the "avoid surgery for back pain" rule. In those cases with severe pain that doesn't respond to activity modification and exercise, surgery to fuse the defect may be indicated. This procedure is more successful that most other back pain surgery because the underlying cause is more straightforward. Certainly, those patients with significant nerve root pinching are good candidates for surgery and usually are much improved after fusion to stabilize the defect.

Ankylosing Spondylitis

This is a rare inflammatory condition of the spine and its ligaments that is related to rheumatoid arthritis. That is to say, it is in that group of diseases we call the "inflammatory joint diseases." This condition leads to a profound stiffening of the spine by causing bone to form in what were once ligaments and discs. It is as if the whole spine from skull to pelvis becomes one petrified bone. "Ankylosis" means to stiffen, and you're now familiar with "spondylo" as in spine. In this case, "spondyl-*itis*" refers to the inflammatory nature of the disease. It is an inflammatory spine disease that leads to stiffening.

Ankylosing spondylitis most commonly affects young men, so it often presents in the boomer age group, first as low back pain. Although this low back pain is associated with an unusual amount of stiffness, don't count on your doctor thinking of this as the first diagnosis. There are plain x-rays (including some of the sacroiliac joints, which are also affected) that make the diagnosis a slam-dunk. But patients who present with this are often misdiagnosed at first and treated for garden-variety back pain.

The treatment for ankylosing spondylitis is similar to the treatment for rheumatoid arthritis: strong drugs directed at relieving inflammation. Patients with this condition are usually under the care of a rheumatologist. From the orthopedic standpoint, the trick is to keep the spine straight, while it's undergoing the inevitable process of fusion. This may involve bracing. You may have seen people walking around with this and didn't know what they had. These are the guys who can't look up, because their spines are fused in a flexed position, sometimes flexed and rotated so they look as if they are always signaling for a right turn.

Coccydynia

Finally, we come to a condition that is truly a "pain in the butt." The coccyx, or "tailbone," is literally a little vestigial tail segment attached at the very end of the spine.

This is one of those little parts that we take for granted until it gets bumped or bruised, often in some totally embarrassing act such as falling flat on your ass. Once pain is incited in this region, it can be very bothersome, chronic and, in some cases, life-altering. Imagine being unable to sit comfortably. Though

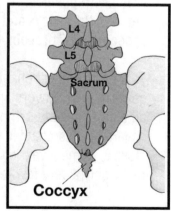

191

the coccyx can be fractured, more commonly it either just bruised badly, or the joint between it and the sacrum above becomes sprained. This condition is more common in women than in men and more common in the skinny than in the heavy patient. It strikes terror in the hearts of doctors. When a skinny woman walks into the office with a little inflatable donut pillow, my heart sinks because I know coccydynia is often recalcitrant to all treatment. It has the reputation of being associated with unusually neurotic patients but I'm not sure this is fair. It may be that it drives people so crazy that by the time they see the doctor they are downright certifiable. Whatever the cause, coccydynia has a bad reputation and most of us flee when we see it coming.

The accepted treatments include padding (the little inflatable donut may not be socially graceful, but it is effective), and various forms of physical therapy, including intra-rectal diathermy, which involves placing a heat probe up the butt. I've always figured that intra-rectal diathermy was like a punitive treatment that doctors prescribed when they wanted to be dead certain that the sufferer would NOT be back. Some surgeons have promoted amputating the coccyx—so-called "coccygectomy"—but I've seen more people who were worse after this than better. I believe the one indication for this radical treatment is a fractured coccyx that has healed in a hooked position. I have sometimes injected the joint between the coccyx and the sacrum with good results. Again, "good results" probably means I didn't see that patient again.

This is the longest chapter for a good reason. Back problems come in many flavors and, collectively, are a big subject with an almost universal impact. I can predict that few of you will have read this chapter without something in it that hit very close to home. I've tried to cover the waterfront, but there are really only a very few recurring themes.

Take care of your back and it is more likely to take care of you. If you have pain from a pinched nerve, surgery can be very helpful; if you have just plain old back pain, surgery is rarely a good idea. If you've gotten into your boomer years without breaking your neck, why risk it now?

Chapter 9: The Hip

You might be surprised to find that what you think of as your hip is probably not the hip I'm going to talk about. When you teach a child to point to her hip, she points to that prominence below the waist and in front of your butt. In fact, your hip joint is in the middle of your groin. "It's in the *crease,* doc," as they would say in New Orleans. But we can't be teaching our kids to go around pointing to the middle of the groin, now can we? As Mammy in *Gone with the Wind* puts it, "Taint fittin'!" So, we grow up thinking that our hip is something way out there in the suburbs, when it is dead center, mid-city. That bump out there you think of as your hip is just a bend in the femur where the muscles that motor the hip attach.

The human hip has to be a sturdy, but mobile joint whose sole purpose in life is the support of bipedal locomotion. The hip is designed for walking upright. It is a deep, constrained, dependable, nothing-fancy ball and socket joint. Unlike the shoulder, it doesn't have a hand attached to it further on down the line, just a lowly foot. It doesn't have to answer to the hand's demand for constant variety, now here, now there. Not that way with the foot. A foot just wants to go forward, always forward. One foot in front of another. One, two, one, two, left, right, left, right, hey, I think I got this down… Oh, there's the occasional sideways gait or maybe the furtive back step, but mostly forward. Fred and Ginger aside, about all the hip has to do is swing the limb forward when the weight is on the opposite hip and then get ready for the impact when it becomes its turn to be the weight-bearing limb. What is amazing is the efficiency of the design of this simple ball in a round hole.

The hip may experience up to five times the body's weight in a typical compressive load, such as running or even getting in or out of a chair. For a two-hundred-pound boomer that means that, at peak loads, his hip weighs in at one half ton. Over time, that joint may wear out. Many of those conditions that present as a failing hip joint in midlife are actually the residuals of some childhood hip problem. The Big Three childhood hip problems are dislocation, the childhood version of osteonecrosis called *Perthes' Disease*, and a condition of growth where the growing, upper end of the femur slips off its moorings. This will require a brief rendition of each condition.

Developmental Dislocation of the Hip

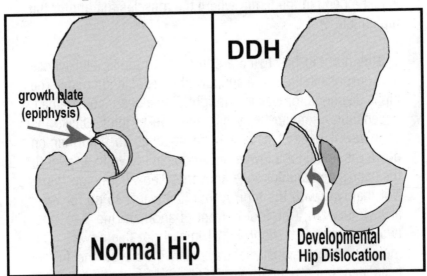

This used to be called "congenital" dislocation but thanks to the lawyers, it now has another name: "developmental" dislocation of the hip. Why the fuss? Because there is a big difference between the two words. Congenital means that the problem was there at the time of birth. Developmental means something that came along some time after birth, during that "developmental" period, as a person's body was growing up.

So, if congenital dislocation means it was there at the time of birth and wasn't recognized, then somebody ought to be liable, right? Somebody must be at fault. It's probably that pediatrician who missed the hip click in the newborn nursery. Or the GP with 500 births under his belt who just missed that one kid's slightly shorter, slightly tighter little leg. Sue him!

But if the condition was "developmental," then it would be expected to show up later. Maybe the child kind of slid into it as he or she began to grow. Or perhaps the hip was just subluxated a little bit at birth, and then, over the first few weeks, went into complete dislocation. You decide, gentle persons of the jury.

Whether you use one term or the other, the truth is that both happen. Many children are born with a dislocated hip. Many others are born with a sloppy hip that's subluxated and on the verge of falling overboard, which, if recognized early, can be treated easily. But if this condition is *not* recognized early and allowed to dislocate completely, these kids may do very poorly or at least require intense treatments, including surgery. The key is not the semantics of the problem, but having an awareness of this condition and screening all kids in the nursery for hip problems.

Hips that have been dislocated in infancy do well if we can get them back into the joint early and keep them there. The development of the hip socket is dependent upon the pressure of the femoral head being in place and on time. If the ball is not directly centered in the socket, the socket will not develop normally, becoming shallow and puny. It may be strong enough to sustain the hip through childhood and adolescence and into young adulthood. But somewhere in the thirties and forties the hip starts to wear out. As with all these types of conditions, the endpoint looks the same: osteoarthritis.

If people with this condition make it into their forties or fifties, many doctors prefer to do a total hip replacement, though some try deepening the socket or redirecting the upper end of the femur. Almost anyway you cut it, if developmental dislocation of the hip comes back to haunt you in your boomer years, chances are you're headed toward some surgical remedy.

Legg-Calve-Perthes Disease

If you have heard of this condition, it is probably because your child has it. This disease occurs during the toddler and early grade school years, or what I think of as the early soccer years. It presents as pain in the groin, in the thigh and often in the knee. Since hip pain is commonly experienced at the knee, it is not unusual for a child with this condition to

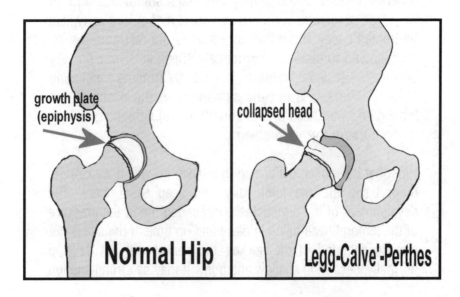

growth plate (epiphysis)

collapsed head

Normal Hip

Legg-Calve'-Perthes

walk around complaining of knee pain. He may have his knee x-rayed several times before someone stumbles onto the notion that, hey, maybe this could be a problem with his hip! What's going on is a peculiar hip condition in which there is a loss of blood supply to the growing femoral head. The ball gets soft and may flatten.

It can affect both hips. The treatment is protective range of motion exercises, bracing and sometimes keeping the hip non-weight-bearing by placing the child on crutches. This solution was at one time taken to extremes. In the 1970s I saw a lecture by a famous British orthopedic surgeon, Ruth Wynn-Davies, who showed pictures of these wards *full* of little children with both legs in casts, the feet spread apart with a broomstick between the ankles, all to keep the hip in position and to keep them from walking. These children spent months in bed. Though this kind of treatment seems barbarous now, the concept was to put the ball into the socket and keep it there while the disease ran its course.

Today we let the children move around but we may use bracing or surgery to accomplish the same thing: keep the hip in the socket while it is undergoing the softening and healing that goes along with this condition. Some children require various surgeries to put the best part of the femoral head back into the socket.

This is another one of those conditions that can get by the censors. I have seen people with the obvious residuals of this condition—-a flattened, shortened femoral head in a congruent oblong socket, formed from the interaction of the deformed femoral head with the developing socket. Although the patient may be having symptoms for the first time in his 40's or 50's, he may remember a period of knee or thigh pain while he was in elementary school. Back then, he was probably told that it was a "groin pull," or "growing pains" or some other such diversion.

Like most childhood problems, this condition heals and the child goes on growing, and rather quickly at that. The worst cases develop problems long before their middle years and require fusion or a hip replacement. Most people with this problem manage to make it into their fifth and sixth decade before they need a hip replacement.

Slipped Capital Femoral Epiphysis (SCFE)

In the bum hip lottery, we have DDH for the newborns, LCPD for the toddlers and little league soccer players, and finally "Slipped Capital Femoral Epiphysis" (SCFE) for the teenagers. This latter condition is just what it sounds like— if you happen to read Latin. It is a slippage (slipped) of the head (capital) of the thigh bone (femoral) at the growth plate (epiphysis). This slippage, the kind that occurs as the ball of the femur slides off its perch on the femoral neck, has been compared to the ice cream melting off and over the end of the cone.

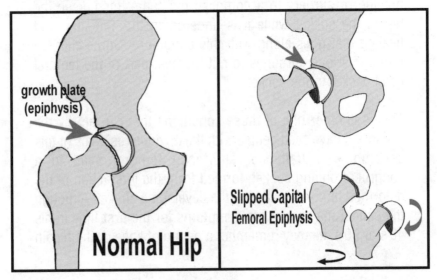

growth plate (epiphysis)

Normal Hip

Slipped Capital Femoral Epiphysis

This condition causes a limp; hip, groin, thigh or knee pain; and often an actual shortening of the leg as it twists outward at the hip.

One way to think of SCFE is as a slow fracture through the growth plate, the disc of cartilage cells from which all future growth is destined to come. Damage the growth plate and you damage growth itself. The trick is to stop the slippage of the ball and, in the worst cases, put it back in place and hold it there surgically.

Almost all SCFEs have to be treated surgically. The treatment is to pin the ball back in place where it should be. A small slippage can be pinned *in situ,* or where it is. Other more displaced cases will need to be reduced or put ever so gently back into place and then pinned to hold them there. The growth plate often stops growing after these slippages occur, but usually there is so little potential for growth left at the hip in this age group that it doesn't matter.

The worst slips, and the ones that go unrecognized, often lead to hip arthritis in the middle years. In this sense this problem is not much different from the other two childhood hip diseases. Any condition that leaves the joint anatomy or mechanics altered will probably lead to arthritis—-though it may take many years.

All three of these childhood hip conditions may lead to what might be called *premature* hip arthritis. If this problem presents in your thirties, it will probably get bad enough that the hip will need replacing in your forties. There is a strong argument in certain cases for a hip fusion. This means completely stiffening the hip by fusing the femur to the pelvis. Remarkably, people function very well with a single hip fusion as long as it is fused in the right position, and as long as there are no other adjacent joints affected. This hip fusion can last forever or can be undone at a later date and converted into a total hip replacement. Having said all that, most patients still look at me like I'm from Mars when I start up this discussion. A fusion is a hard operation to sell, especially now that total hip replacement is available.

Total Hip Replacement

I began this discussion in *Chapter 3, Arthritis*, so some of this will be repetition, but here I will go into more detail. You met the inventor, Dr. John Charnley and read about the development of this procedure. So where are we now with hip replacement? What are the common indications in the boomer patient?

The most common indications for hip replacement in

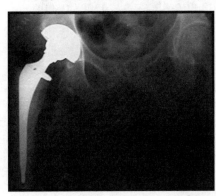

the boomer age group is osteoarthritis, sometimes with a definable antecedent among the childhood hip diseases (dislocation, Legg-Calve-Perthes Disease or slipped capital femoral epiphysis), trauma or just early onset arthritis on an inherited basis.

There are some new developments on the horizon for hip replacement, particularly as regards new types of bearing surfaces. Most total hips loosen over time because of what we doctors call "the cellular events stimulated by the generation of polyethylene wear debris." Stick with me now, this is easier than it sounds. In plain English, God didn't give us any cells or enzymes to digest plastic. As the implanted artificial hip joint is loaded around one million times per year, there is bound to be some wear debris generated from the metal head moving against the plastic socket. This debris, actually little particles of polyethylene, incites a response from the cells that are supposed to be on KP duty. These garbage collectors arrive on the scene and throw their best stuff at these particles, but they cannot get rid of this plastic debris. They try every enzyme "digestase" that they have in their arsenal, but there just is no "polyethylene-ase" that will dissolve it. Unfortunately, in their exuberant attempts to digest the plastic, they do succeed in digesting a good bit of the adjacent bone. This weakens the bone and its bond to the prosthesis. It doesn't matter whether that bond is bone cement or a prosthesis held in place by bone-ingrowth into the prosthesis. The same process can loosen either.

The quest for the life-lasting hip replacement has become an Argosy in search not of the Golden Fleece, but rather the Perfect Bearing Surface. If we could find new materials that both did the job and generated little or no wear debris, then we might get these suckers to last a long, long time. Right now that search has focused on metal-on-metal bearings and ceramic bearings. The problem here is that in joint replacement, we just don't what will turn out to be a bad idea until about five to ten years into the replacement when things start to show signs that they may auger in[12]. Conservative surgeon that I am, I will wait for those pioneers to work out the bugs. But we do make certain concessions and modifications when performing hip replacement on young people. We usually use un-cemented, bone-ingrowth components, avoiding cement. In some younger patients I will use a ceramic, actually zirconium, prosthetic head. These ultra-smooth and ultra-hard heads reduce the friction against the polyethylene, and should significantly reduce the wear debris, hopefully prolonging the life of the prosthesis. The

12 This is USAF jargon for anything gone really bad. It alludes to the path a downed plane makes as it crashes.

trade off is that these advanced bearing surfaces are pricey, almost doubling the cost of a hip replacement. I think this is well justified in the young patient and not necessary in the average elderly, lower-demand patient.

Probably the most exciting recent advance in hip replacement is the improvement in the polyethylene (plastic) itself. In the last several years, the wear characteristics have been so enhanced that laboratory testing suggests we may have significantly reduced the wear that leads to the loosening. We are already using these new polyethylene bearings routinely, and we should know soon if they prove to be as good in the human body as they seem to be in the laboratory.

There is another very recent trend toward doing hip replacements through ever smaller incisions. These are (I think) mistakenly called "minimally invasive" procedures. To my way of thinking, there's nothing minimally invasive about cutting out the femoral head, reaming out the socket and replacing the whole joint with metal and plastic—no matter how small the incision. I openly discuss my conservative surgical bias in the last chapter, *Chapter 15: the Paradoxes.* Here I advise patients to be careful. This new wrinkle in a very successful operation may seem attractive, but I'm not convinced it offers significant advantages. But I guarantee that it will be heavily marketed. In the worst case scenario you might hook up with a surgeon who is at the beginning of what is a steep learning curve and be trading more problems for a smaller incision.

Fractures

If you think of hip fractures as something that happens to frail old people, by and large, you are right. For these poor old folks, a fall from ground height will shatter their brittle skeleton. The robust boomer would take that fall and bounce up for a backhand crosscourt winner. It takes a lot more kinetic energy to break the normal hip. In vehicular mayhem, or a fall from a great height, both of which are considered "recreational pursuits" by some boomers, some of the most serious injuries involve fracturing the strong protective pelvis itself. Second only to the Brain in sturdy self preservation, the thick bones of the pelvis are designed to resist the stresses of running and jumping, though not running into things or trying to jump through things. Pelvic fractures are often life-threatening injuries that can render a patient dead at the scene of the crime from sheer blood loss. Many DOAs[13] have this. A good number of patients who don't make it to the Emergency Room or die en route, die of blood loss from massive pelvic trauma. The pelvis is a very sturdy structure and it takes a near lethal amount of energy to breach its defenses. But once disrupted, the large vessels protected by the pelvic bones may tear, producing a disastrous hemorrhage that simply cannot be controlled.

When the pelvis doesn't fracture, sometimes the upper end of the femur will break against it. When the Brain sees a hip fracture coming, it orders "STOP!" sending out an urgent order for all limbs, uppers and lowers, to shoot out STRAIGHT, right now! The seated driver instantly assumes the terrified defensive position, both legs out straight, slamming on the brakes, both arms out straight, a death grip on the wheel. If he's lucky, he gets slammed in the face with a big airbag, but maybe not before his right leg has locked on that brake pedal at the same moment that the floorboards are being driven up into said brake pedal, forcing the lower extremity violently back in line with itself, shattering the femur at the hip.

13 "DOA" = dead on arrival.

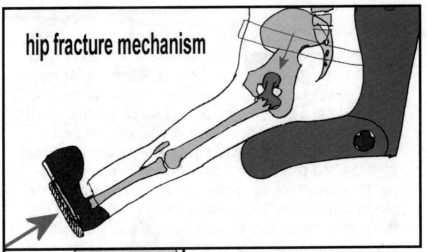

hip fracture mechanism

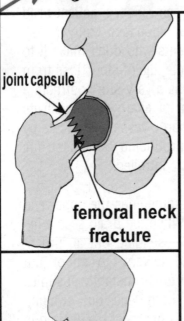

joint capsule

femoral neck fracture

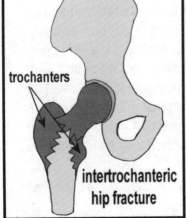

trochanters

intertrochanteric hip fracture

That's how we baby boomers get ours. Not from some fall on the way to dinner. No. We go down in big, ugly tangles of metal and glass bits all over. Or we fall from the roof while putting up the satellite dish. Two stories ought to do it. Or we fly off that bicycle careening down the hill *with the wind in our hair.* "Oh no, Mr. Bill! Not a broken hip!"

Although it takes a lot more force to make them happen, most hip fractures in the boomer age group fall into the same general categories as those in the elderly. The two most common breaks are those inside the joint along the femoral neck and those that occur at the bend in the femur below the hip joint where the large muscles are attached. The first are called "femoral neck fractures" and the second are called "intertrochanteric fractures," since they occur between the two bumps called trochanters.

Intertrochanteric fractures can be fixed with plates and screws and can be expected to heal fairly well. Femoral neck fractures are prone to all sorts of problems. A displaced femoral neck fracture in a forty year-old is a scary situation. The chances are higher that there will be either a failure of healing (non-union) or a collapse of the ball from the loss of blood supply, or osteonecrosis.

We've encountered this concept of osteonecrosis before when discussing fractures of the scaphoid. Here is another example of a bone with a stranded blood supply, much like a light bulb completely enclosed in the socket, with its sole sustaining supply of electricity coming into it only through the filament end. The blood supply to the femoral head courses up along the neck of the femur from a ring of blood vessels that circles its base. Break the neck and you interrupt the blood supply, just like cutting your own neck would shut off the blood supply to your brain. Osteonecrosis ("dead bone") is the softening and collapse that occurs in the femoral head when it tries to heal the break. Sometimes the fracture may heal and the patient and surgeon rejoice at having dodged the first bullet, only to be shot down by the late onset of osteonecrosis, a year or two later.

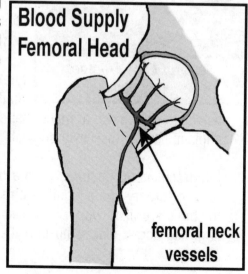

Blood Supply Femoral Head

femoral neck vessels

Femoral neck fractures are treated surgically with a closed reduction—meaning the fracture is set by pulling on the leg in the right direction—then secured in place with long screws that go up from the outside of the intact femur into the fractured head. Since this is a somewhat precarious fixation at best, the patient is not allowed to put weight on this construct until healing can be seen. This usually means at least six weeks on crutches, not touching the foot to the ground, or what we cleverly call "non-weight-bearing," and then another few months of gradually putting more weight across it as it heals. Laborers can be out for six months with one of these injuries—easy. If you add up the incidence of osteonecrosis and add to that the incidence of failed healing, in a young person you have a less than fifty-fifty chance of getting a good result with a displaced fracture. In old folks, we just throw the head away and replace it with a metal one.

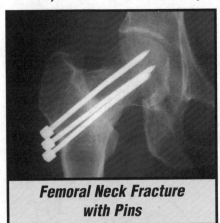

Femoral Neck Fracture with Pins

That will last the few years they have left on the planet, but is just not acceptable for the young and pathologically active. Here, we pin even the most displaced injury and hope for the best. This choice doesn't burn any bridges and, if it falls apart, we can always go on to a total hip replacement. Those that heal and don't get osteonecrosis have a much better hip, than any I can implant, namely their own original.

Intertrochanteric fractures have a better prognosis but still require surgery and a significant recuperative period. These fractures are fixed with a so-called "compression screw," a large lag screw placed up into the femoral head from the

inside, then secured to a
barrel plate that is itself
screwed onto the shaft of
the bone, along the side
of the femur. Now we're
talking serious hardware.
These fractures usually heal
quickly and solidly and are
not prone to the same
circulatory embarrassment
as their cousins at the

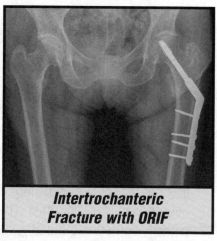

**Intertrochanteric
Fracture with ORIF**

femoral neck. However, the damage done to the large muscle
attachments can subtly rearrange the mechanics of the hip,
leaving the boomer with a limp.

Traumatic hip dislocations do occur but, like fractures, they
really require a lot of force. Once again, we see these
dislocations only after a vehicular trauma or a fall from a
ridiculous height. Skiing is actually right up there with those
other "mechanisms of injury," as we blithely call them.
Anything that forces the flexed knee out against some
immovable object will likely force the hip either out the back

of the socket or worse yet,
through it. These very violent
injuries are often associated
with fractures of either the
femoral head and neck, or
fractures of the socket itself.
Here the risk of osteonecrosis
is very high because the
dislocation may wrench away
the circulation to the head,
stripping off its blood supply.
These are surgical emergencies
in which every effort should be

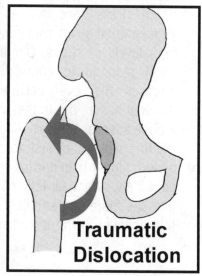

**Traumatic
Dislocation**

made to get the dislocated head reduced and back into the socket as soon as possible.

The orthopod will usually ask the general surgeon to stand aside while he just "pops this in," before the belly surgeon whisks the patient away to the OR to stop the bleeding liver and patch up the other perforated organs. Reducing a dislocated hip involves two strong people. One stands astride the pelvis, pushing down with both hands as a counterweight. The other (the surgeon) stands over the patient, sometimes literally standing on the gurney, pulling with all his might on the leg with the knee flexed. He cradles the poor soul's leg in his arms while yanking upwards toward the ceiling, twisting as he does. CluuuunnnnnK! "It's back in. You can go save his life now. We have saved his hip."

Stress Fractures

Boomers have plenty of stress. I'm not talking about the psychological kind here, but what engineers mean by stress: the application of force per unit area. If you have a lot of a force, such as the force of squeezing that we call "compression," spread out over a large area, there won't be much stress generated. If you have a fairly small force concentrated on an even smaller area, you can achieve pretty high levels of stress. Our bones get in trouble when they must respond to cumulative stress. Bones like normal stresses; they even need them to stay strong. But every material has a limit to the amount of stress it can absorb. If a bone absorbs stress suddenly during a vehicular trauma, a fracture will occur, just as suddenly. If a bone is forced to absorb higher than normal stresses repetitively, it will fail just as surely. We call this condition a "stress fracture" or, perhaps more appropriately, "fatigue fracture." I introduced this concept in the last chapter, referring to spondylolysis.

Fatigue fractures are usually heralded by a slow onset of pain in a particular region, in this case the groin. These stress fractures are common throughout the lower extremity.

Stress fractures of the hip are high risk for the same reason as other femoral neck fractures. Namely, if they displace they may lead to either non-union or osteonecrosis. Yet, these fractures never just come out of the blue. There is usually at least a week or two of "prodrome," a sort of physical premonition with hip pain after exercise. In the case of military recruits, this "exercise" is supervised by a big ugly drill sergeant who would like nothing better than to see you cave in. Only three animals get stress fractures: race horses, race dogs and human beings. We three are the only animals loyal enough or dumb enough to run 'til we break.

In boomers, these fatigue fractures of the hip are almost always going to present after some recent increase in physical activity. Suddenly, after almost 40 years, John Kennedy's moving words about what a bunch of slobs we were getting to be finally kicks in. Maybe you buy that Tae Bo video. Now you're dancing and bouncing and throwing sloppy punches at your own private Lester Spinks and, ouch, got a little pain in the crease here, doc. Probably just a "groin pull." No pain, no gain. Bounce, kick, punch, "Yo! That ain't no groin pull. Where's that phone book?"

You can see this condition across all the Syndromes. The deconditioned, sadly, get it trying to make up for years of inactivity. The jocks overdo it training for that marathon or that Iron Man. Narcissus squats way too much weight trying to push his thighs from the Volkswagen to the Rolls Royce category. Finally, the used-to-be-a-fat-lady does it all too often, trying to put ever more distance between her skinny, underfed, anorexic, amenorrheic self and that chubby little girl waddling along behind, ready to catch her. The key is to be aware of the diagnosis. Get to your doctor if you have persistent pain in the groin or thigh after exercise. A simple x-ray is often enough, and when it isn't, either an MRI or a bone scan will settle the question. And it is a big question, because if the problem is, in fact, a stress fracture of the hip, it should be prophylactically pinned to prevent displacement and promote healing. If this goes un-recognized or gets blown off as something less, disaster can strike.

Groin Muscle Pulls

I mention this only to emphasize that this is what we call a "diagnosis of exclusion." This means that you don't call an injury a "groin pull" until you've eliminated everything else that it might be. When the patient comes in with pain in the groin and thigh, particularly after exercise or as a problem they've developed slowly, I don't jump to the diagnosis of a pulled muscle. I have to prove to myself first that it's not a stress fracture, an early presentation of arthritis, or even a referred pain from the back. This is like the example of the "sprained wrist" you should be unwilling to diagnose until your doctor has ruled out a fractured scaphoid. People do pull groin muscles with crazy stunts like splits or unexpected stunts like falls and even intentional stunts like team sports, but you have to exclude the painted horses before you call this one a zebra.

You don't want this diagnosis anyway, because they take forever to heal and often lead to prolonged pain with physical activity. There is little or no treatment other than stretching and gradual re-strengthening.

Snapping Hip Syndrome

This unusual condition is almost exclusively seen in

Snapping Hip Syndrome

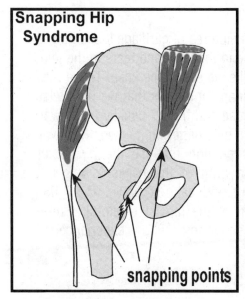

snapping points

women and may have a number of causes. We have to round up the usual suspects of things that go "bump in the night." In the case of things that can snap around the hip, we have intra-articular causes (things loose in the joint) and extra-articular causes (things that snap over the moving joint).

Patients with this problem usually experience a painful snapping or popping over the side or the front of the hip, often with flexion. This symptom may be consistent, but more often it is unpredictable and adheres to the old adage, "It'll never do it when I go to the doctor's." This problem is really hard to sort out and notoriously difficult to treat. The most common snappers are the tendons that flex the hip and the large ligament that stretches over the outside of it.

These can be stretched with therapy or even surgically lengthened, but this type of surgery is fairly high risk and low yield.

The loose-things-in-the-joint category sounds like it would be easier to recognize and easier to treat, but actually the things that cause it are extremely difficult to visualize even with an MRI. There are only a few surgeons in the country heroic enough to routinely stick the arthroscope into the hip. Unlike the knee which is very accessible to the arthroscope, and which has a large potential space in which to maneuver, the hip is deep, tight and less accessible. But those few hip arthroscopists have gotten pictures of cartilage loose bodies similar to the debris we see in the knee and tears in the joint ligaments—again, much like we see in the knee. These may account for some of the snaps and pops that we otherwise have been unable to diagnose and treat. I usually try to wait this condition out to see if it gets better on its own. But I will sometimes be suspicious enough that it's the hip flexor muscle snapping over the brim of the pelvis to inject it with x-ray guidance to try and calm it down. If all this doesn't work and the MRI of the hip isn't helpful, I refer the patient to another surgeon in town who is experienced at hip arthroscopy.

Trochanteric Bursitis

Finally, we come to something common and usually treatable, the condition we call trochanteric bursitis. This is a pain over the outside of the hip, actually right in that place where the child points when you ask, "Where's your hip, Shawna?" We've already encountered the term "trochanter" before. Recall that it is that prominence where the hip bone bends and some of the large muscle of ambulation are attached. At times, we experience pain at this friction surface, which may make it painful to sit up, get up or to lie on that hip at night.

Large forces are at play here. We call this condition a bursitis because then we try to blame pain in that region on an inflammation of the bursa that lies over the trochanter, hence the term "trochanteric bursitis." Here I'm a non-traditionalist. I've opened thousands of hips over the past 28 years and have seen only a few inflamed bursae. Those were in conditions known to be primarily inflammatory in nature— rheumatoid arthritis, say. What we call trochanteric bursitis, I think is actually a muscle insertion problem. When it occurs in the elbow, it's called epicondylitis. When it occurs in the shoulder, we know it as rotator cuff tendonitis. In the hip we could call it "trochanteritis", I suppose, but the term trochanteric bursitis has stuck.

I say this not to confuse you, but just to explain that many of the middle-aged folks whom I see for this diagnosis have associated back problems. These may refer pain into the hip area or may cause weakness in the muscles that attach there. Many times, if you don't also treat the adjacent back problem, you can't help the patient's hip pain symptoms disappear.

In the end, no matter what you choose to call this problem, we treat it first with NSAIDs (ibuprofen and similar drugs) and stretching and, finally, with cortisone shots, presumably into the ailing bursa, but actually in the general direction of the painful muscle insertion. This condition is chronic by nature and may persist for months at a time. It may or may not respond to shots. Though there are surgical procedures recommended for this, I can truthfully say that I've never seen fit to employ any. This is one of the conditions from which we get the slang, "pain in the butt."

Though I've wandered in this chapter from childhood to senescence, and from some very serious conditions to less serious ones, I'd like to close by talking once again about total hip replacement and my hero, Dr. John Charnley. We've seen that boomer hip problems can represent the residuals of childhood hip troubles, de novo osteoarthritis, acute fractures, more chronic stress fractures, or the usual gamut of tendonitis and muscle injuries that can afflict almost any joint. Because the hip is so central to gait, almost none of these problems can be ignored. Prior to the 1960s and Dr. Charnley, the inventor of modern total hip replacement, patients with severe hip arthritis were condemned to live out their lives with a painful limp, on a cane or even crutches. His operation is truly one of the greatest advancements of twentieth century medicine. To anyone who has had a successful hip replacement, this is no overstatement. Of all the procedures I do, this one helps more people, more consistently than any other. It can take a wheelchair-bound patient and get him back on his feet, often walking without a cane. It is a Lazarus operation if there ever was one. Many of the serious problems that I've just described eventually lead to end-stage osteoarthritis of the hip, which we treat with total hip replacement. Though we take it for granted, this is as close to a miracle as anything I do.

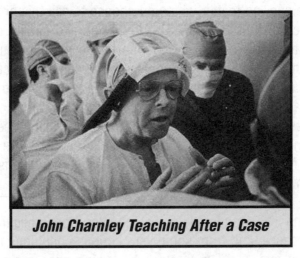

John Charnley Teaching After a Case

Chapter 10: The Knee

The knee is the most common area of complaint I see in my boomer patients, followed closely by the shoulder. Since the knee is often injured during athletics, most of you probably have a friend or two who tore up their knees in high school or college.

When we were in school in the 50's, 60's and 70's, the science of repairing the damaged knee was rudimentary. Even the basic understanding of the biomechanics of the knee and how it worked was in its infancy when I was undergoing my training at Mayo's in the 1970's. Much of what we now understand about the knee grew out of the technological advancements that came with total knee replacement and arthroscopic surgery. This is analogous to the space program where NASA had to push out the envelope of science to meet the technological demands of the race to put a man on the moon. In the case of the knee, we started with a simplistic concept that it was basically a hinge. So when we first tried to replace it, our artificial joints looked like a hinge. They failed miserably because the knee is a much more sophisticated gliding, sliding, rotating mechanism. Any hinge that didn't account for all that gliding and sliding and rotating was doomed to failure. And so was your knee if you happened to tear it up before we understood all that.

Arthritis

In the clinic I see a lot of men and women my age who have long, ugly scars up and down either side of the knee, usually from the operations we did at the time to cut out torn cartilages. These were open amputations of the damaged part. Since the little rubbery cartilages we call the "menisci" are there for a reason, cutting the whole thing out might be expected to have long-term side effects. In this case the end result is arthritis. But in order to make sense of that, I'll have to pause here and review what we mean by arthritis. It just so happens that the knee is an excellent joint to illustrate this point.

As you learned in *Chapter 3*, arthritis is not just some mild achy pain that they use to sell Tylenol (acetaminophen) on the evening news. It's not just a little stiffness that you get when the weather changes. Osteoarthritis is the final common pathway for a whole bunch of conditions, but in the end they result in failure of that organ we call the joint.

I've spent a large part of my career explaining to people that arthritis is not just something minor that comes and goes away with ibuprofen. In fact, it's the reason that we do all these joint replacements, upwards of 250,000 each of total hip and total knee replacements every year in this country. That figure will only rise as our bulge in the python matures and continues to cause us to suffer the ravages of damage to these major weight-bearing joints. I just saw the statistics from my own practice, and this year the three of us that do joint replacements have done well over four hundred among us. About two thirds of those are knees and the other third are hips, and a smaller number of shoulders. Arthritis of the knee is serious business.

The crowd that I see in my office falls roughly into three categories. First, I'll discuss those who already have advanced arthritis of the knee from some injury in our reckless youth. In these cases there is little to do but wait it out until the condition is disabling enough to have the knee replaced. Though there is no lower age limit to knee replacement, we have to understand that these implants are artificial constructs, implanted into a hostile environment (the human boomer body) and will only deteriorate over time. So we encourage people to wait as long as they reasonably can. Even here we've changed our attitude over the last twenty years. We now feel that it is better to offer a forty-five-year-old a total knee replacement, if he otherwise meets the indications for surgery, rather than make him wait until some arbitrary age like, say, sixty-five. Everyone is happier if he has his pain relief and increased function during his productive years, than if he limps around for twenty years, and then enjoys his retirement. We are also better able to revise implants that have worn or loosened after a ten, fifteen or twenty year lifetime.

Sore Kneecaps

The second category I see is the women (and a few men) with sore kneecaps. This condition causes pain in the front of the knee, usually worse with things that stress the kneecap (patella) such as stair climbing, squatting, kneeling etc. This has a host of aliases, the most common of which is "chondromalacia patella," literally "cartilage illness of the kneecap." This condition is more common in women because of the variance in normal gender anatomy that makes their hips wider than men's, often creating a greater angle against which the female's patella must pull when it works to straighten the knee. The patella is just a bone in the tendon of the big muscle in the front of the thigh, the muscle called the quadriceps. This muscle pulls to straighten the knee, arresting that reciprocal, controlled falling-forward motion that we call "walking." As the quad contracts, it pulls the patella against the femur where it glides through a groove in the front of the knee.

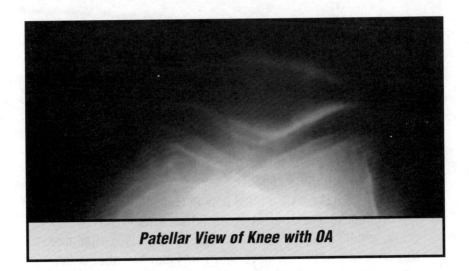

Patellar View of Knee with OA

This groove and its depth and direction are one of the unique features of those primates that have assumed an upright posture. This is what those anthropologists are looking at in an early hominid like "Lucy" when they conclude that she was a walker.

This special articulation generates huge stresses when you squat or walk up or down stairs. In fact, these stresses can rise to over five times your body weight. If you weigh two-hundred pounds, that amounts to around a half ton of compressive load on the kneecap. ("What did the doctor say?" Tearfully, "He said I weighed half a ton!") So now, lets get on that StairMaster and do a few thousand flights! Not good? Well, then lets go to step aerobics class and burn off a few cartilage cells. You see my point.

This is clearly not a condition requiring surgery. It is knee pain caused by an overload, and the treatment for an overload is to remove the stressful condition that is precipitating it, if you can. Treadmill walking without much incline is a good substitute for knee-destroying exercises like stair-stepping because the knees are not loaded by bending them as much. You can still put on the leotards, the Walkman, the little water bottle and the whole bit. Avoid well-intentioned arthroscopic surgery! Lots of quick fixes have been described by doctors but, by and large, the patient who has some anatomic abnormality that can be remedied with the knife is the exception. Isometric quadriceps strengthening, hamstring stretching, ice and avoiding the things that got you into this situation are still the mainstays of treatment for sore kneecaps.

In my practice I have frequently seen the young woman in her mid thirties who comes to me for treatment of a chronic knee problem. Her situation illustrates how the over-aggressive treatment of patellofemoral problems can have disastrous results. I'll call my composite patient Paula, as in "the Perils of Paula's Patella."

Paula developed pain in the kneecap in her teenage years as is true of so many active, athletic young women. First her doctor tried a brief course of injections and some physical therapy. He also tried to get her to limit the activities that worsened the problem. Paula had problems with both knees, but the right one was worse, so it got most of the attention. Eventually, this "attention" included an arthroscopic surgery to scrape the cartilage on the underside of the patella. That didn't help. Next, they tried a lateral release procedure, which meant cutting the "tight" reigns on the lateral side of the patella so that it would "track better." I put these terms in quotes, because I'm certain that Paula had nothing really wrong with her patellar tracking or with tight ligaments on the lateral side. The lateral release actually made her worse. So next they tried a more aggressive realignment procedure in which the whole patellar ligament was lifted up and screwed back down a little to one side, again with the idea of improving the patellar tracking. Once again, things actually got worse and now the pain was so bad and her muscles so weak that she was constantly on crutches, and in terrible pain. Eventually, the surgeons resorted to that ultimate solution for the painful anything: ablation. They did a "patellectomy"—they cut out the patella. All this well-intentioned surgery tied up a good part of her late teens and her early twenties.

After the patellectomy, Paula got some improvement for a few years. Then in her early thirties, she began to develop the inevitable osteoarthritis. When she first came to see me, she had frank osteoarthritis. We've been working together for years now. I've mainly injected the knee now and then, cleaned out (with the arthroscope) some of the worst junk from the arthritis and helped prepare her for the eventual total knee replacement.

What ever happened with the other knee? As is almost always the case, the knee that had no surgery is the best one. The one that was the beneficiary of all those modern surgical interventions is a worn-out, painful mess. Worse yet, when I finally do that total knee, she will not function quite as well as a patient who still has a patella. I can't put that bone back, and I can't resurface it if it's not there. Whenever I see some young woman in the office who thinks she's at the end of her rope with this kneecap pain and who is crying out for surgery, I emphasize the importance of the therapeutic exercises, avoiding the activities that bother the knee, and avoiding surgery, however well-intentioned. And sometimes I have them call Paula. She's very willing to tell her story to anyone I refer to her.

Worn-out Cartilage

In *Chapter 3: Arthritis* I discussed the arthritic knee, worn out cartilage and the role of arthroscopic surgery in each. Remember the Parable of the Laborer and the Lawyer? No need to repeat it here, but if you want to review that section, it is on pages 61-64. Just to review the basic concept, the arthroscope is fine for taking out meniscus cartilage and not good at doing anything for arthritis. As yet we can't "re-plaster the roof" or repair the articular cartilage when it's wearing out. The most common condition I see in boomers is a degenerative tear of the back part of the medial meniscus, causing pain and mechanical symptoms. As long as there is no or at least not much associated arthritis (wear and tear of the articular cartilage surface), then arthroscopic removal of the worn out portion of the meniscus is usually very effective…at least in the short term. But make no mistake about it, this is knee that is starting to wear out.

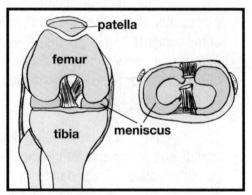

I discussed knee replacement in *Chapter 3: Arthritis*. It has now become one of the most common operations that we do. Though this used to be an operation reserved for the elderly, we now often perform knee replacements in midlife. We expect at least 90% survival of these implants at 10 years and many go 15 years. I let my knee replacement patients golf, but not play tennis. I ask them to avoid running, jumping or twisting activities. After all, we need to remind ourselves that this is an artificial implant, made of metal and plastic and though it is marvelous at relieving knee pain while walking, it cannot simulate normal knee mechanics or durability. Walk all you want, but don't let me catch you water-skiing.

The usual hospitalization for a knee replacement is three to five days, but the rehab lasts for several months. I tell patients to expect at least a three month recovery. A guy with a sit-down job might be back at work in a month, but the guy who has to climb or walk long distances should tell his boss he won't be in for at least three months.

Total knees function well, but almost never have the full flexion (bending) that a normal knee has. This limits people with jobs that require squatting, or getting down into low places. Knee replacements don't kneel very well, either. I find some patients can kneel just fine, but the majority are not comfortable kneeling on the operated knee. This also has implications for the boomer whose job involves getting down on his knees.

The biggest issue with doing knee replacements in the midlife age group is making sure that everyone—patient and physician alike—understands that this will ultimately need revision surgery. Hopefully this second operation will be ten or fifteen years down the line, and I would rather give a 50 year-old patient that time with a pain-free knee, than make him wait until he's some arbitrary age. We should accept the inevitability of revision and get on with it.

Trauma: Torn Ligaments and Damaged Pride

The first three conditions I've discussed represent the majority of the non-traumatic knee complaints I see. These are the insidious, slow-onset, nagging things that sneak up on you, gradually get worse and finally require attention. But boomers are too ambitious, too energetic to leave it at that. Pride goeth before the fall. They think they should be able to saunter into a tangle of twenty-year-old college dropouts for a little game of pick up hoops. Hey, who gets the balding, gray-haired honkey guy? Yep, or better yet, he'll go over the edge on that black diamond slope thinking "I used to be really good at this…man, *feel the wind in my hair!*" Splaat! Boomers seem to want to be felled by something more glamorous that just arthritis. Old people get arthritis; a boomer tears up his knee when he dumps his bike in the Iron Man.

Some of the most severely disabling injures are to the knee ligaments, an intricate arrangement of strong restraining straps. These allow the knee not only to flex and extend as if it were a simple hinge, but also to rotate and translate slightly. They provide just enough of this slipping around to accommodate moving over uneven ground, cutting and going sideways, presenting the foot to the ground at all sorts of different knee angles etc. When we engage in any sport or activity that involves a lot of jumping, starting and stopping, and cutting and going, we are at risk to tear a knee ligament. If you throw in the controlled chaos of a football field, a soccer pitch or a basketball court, it should come as no surprise that knee ligaments are frequently injured in these sports. We call these injuries "sprains." As you will recall, a sprain is an injury to a ligament. A "strain" is an injury to a musculo-tendinous unit (as in muscles or their tendons).

These ligament sprains may vary from a mild stretch that causes pain but no instability, to a complete rupture. Complete rupture of any ligament usually means that the ligament can no longer do its job. Whatever it was supposed to hold together is going to be looser from now on. In the knee there are two main pairs of ligaments: the two along the sides called "collateral ligaments" and another pair in the center that cross, called the "cruciate ligaments." These ligaments all work together to keep the knee going in the right direction without too much play in this direction or that. A sudden excessive force, such as that inflicted by a defensive lineman rolling up onto an offensive lineman's leg, can stress the ligament beyond failure and it will rupture— either tear in the middle or avulse itself from one of its bony anchors. Either way there is bleeding, swelling, pain and consternation. If the ligament is completely torn, a person may also experience instability, as the joint is suddenly without one of its restraints.

Collateral ligament injuries are less severe than cruciate ligament injuries. They may be just as painful but, in general, they heal with bracing and only occasionally need surgery. On the contrary, cruciate ligament injuries just don't heal. This has to do with their being inside the joint, bathed in joint fluid, and other reasons having to do with the blood supply. Once they are torn, they remain torn. We can sew the ends back together, but they still don't heal. Cruciate ligaments behave like brain tissue: the damage is permanent.

The most famous of all these injuries is the sprain of the anterior cruciate ligament. This is the dreaded "ACL Tear." This injury commonly occurs as a so-called "non-contact" injury, where the patient goes up wrong, comes

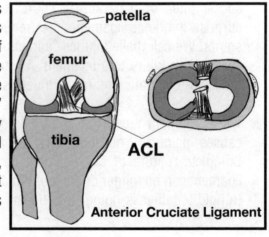

down wrong, cuts wrong or otherwise jigs when his ACL thought he was supposed to jag. The ACL controls the knee's subtle rotation, as well as the movement of the tibia forward on the femur. The knee has about twenty-five or thirty degrees of rotation that normally a simple hinge couldn't have. Ah, but simple hinges can't do reverse slam-dunks, now can they? Simple hinges can't sprint forward through a line of ravenous, over-heated, three hundred-pound men, then plant and go just as suddenly sideways at ninety degrees off the first path. Knees can do that. Young knees can do that some of the time. Older, maturing, more experienced knees ought to know better. But apparently they don't, because I see a bunch of boomers limping in with painful swollen knees and a story that starts, "Well, Doc, we were playing one-on-one… I don't know, he was probably twenty-four, twenty-five max…when I came down off this rebound wrong and heard a pop."

That "pop" is the last gasp of the ACL as it is twisted into oblivion. After rupturing, it begins bleeding into the joint, rather rapidly filling it with blood, making what may have seemed a surprisingly minor injury into a painful swollen knee. Unfortunately, that's the common denominator with knee injuries: a painful, swollen knee. A day or two after the initial injury, they all look remarkably alike. If one has the privilege of examining these injuries immediately after they occur—such as the team doc who sprints out onto the field and puts the knee through its paces before the John Deer with the stretcher on it gets there—you can get a surprisingly good idea of what the damage is. Once the pain and spasm set in, however, a painful, swollen knee can be very hard to examine and hard on the patient if you don't do it right.

I've joked in these pages about orthopods performing a physical exam sprinkled with provocative maneuvers designed to make the diagnosis by eliciting pain. In reality, we try pretty hard to avoid unnecessary pain or discomfort to the patient being examined. Nowhere is eliciting pain more counter-productive than when examining the painful, swollen, recently injured knee. If the patient can't relax some, the surgeon will never be able to tell by his exam if a ligament may be torn. Many times, the diagnosis can be made by taking the history of the injury and performing the physical exam, but not always. If the exam is non-specific, we get an MRI, which is an excellent tool for diagnosing ligament injuries and often a big help in planning the treatment. In fact, in current practice, it is routine to get an MRI for all but the most benign appearing knee injuries.

The surgical repair of a ruptured ACL is actually a surgical reconstruction of the ligament done by substituting either a thick piece of the kneecap tendon or a doubled-up length of the hamstring tendons. This is big surgery that takes a long time to get over. This type of athlete goes down on the field, gets carted off on the John Deer with the stretcher, has the MRI on Monday, gets his knee reconstructed on Wednesday and is out for the season. Maybe he never is

quite the athlete he was before he tore his ACL.

Not every fifty-year-old boomer should get his ACL reconstructed. Here's how I sort them out. Some people have loose joints, as we saw in the case of the

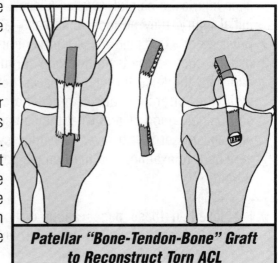

Patellar "Bone-Tendon-Bone" Graft to Reconstruct Torn ACL

shoulder. Some people have stiffer joints with tighter ligaments. When the knee loses its ACL, how well it functions depends a lot on the inherent stability of what's left. Some knees just have better, tighter restraints than others. Those loosey-goosey knees with an extra ten or fifteen degrees of extension cannot be expected to do well when they lose the ACL. For this reason, after the same injury, some people get along better than others.

In fact, there are plenty of people running around out there with an old torn ACL. Those that get along well usually limit their participation in cutting and turning sports, and learn to live with the minor instability. Others with looser knees may find that they have instability while performing everyday activities. They get out of the chair and their knee gives way. They turn the corner on the street and the knee buckles. No matter what they do, the knee has become unpredictable and undependable. Then finally, there are those who only experience instability episodes when they try to resume cutting sports. They can jog and treadmill and all that, but they can't play basketball or soccer with the kids.

Those who are stable enough that they have no daily misery with this condition we leave alone. Those who have clear-cut instability during activities of daily living need to be reconstructed. Those two endpoints are simple. The decision is harder for the middle ground: patients with occasional episodes and those that are not happy to live life without the competition that they should have given up a long time ago. Here the surgeon and the patient need to have a long talk exploring the tradeoffs between living with reality, maybe modifying a few behaviors, and a big surgery that takes a long time to get over. The results of ACL reconstruction are generally very good but, like all operations, it is certainly not without complications. The surgeon and the patient have to make an informed decision together.

It's important to note that a reconstructed ligament is not "as good as new" or (I've heard this a lot) "stronger than the one I tore." Nope, it's still a compromise, using some other tissue to substitute for one of the most sophisticated ligaments in the body. There is no way it could ever be the same. And guess what? It's a seriously damaged knee, reconstructed or not. The chances of developing later osteoarthritis are significantly higher than for a knee that was never injured. With luck the patient gets a stable knee with little loss of motion and good relief from pain. With luck, the surgeon is able to educate the patient and convince him to consider taking inventory of all the unnecessary physical challenges he may be presenting to this newly reconstructed knee.

Fractures Around the Knee

Luckily, fractures involving the knee are not common in boomers. But two injuries occur commonly enough to deserve discussion: fractures of the kneecap and fractures of the tibia plateau.

In the last chapter on the hip, I gave a description of the last few nanoseconds before our hero crashes his Lexus. Imagine that he has a late deployment of that airbag and his flexed knee is smashed against the dash. The first thing to fracture is the first thing to make direct contact: the patella. For this reason, patellar fractures are commonly caused by motor vehicle accidents or any fall onto the flexed knee. The patella is driven deep into the groove in the femur in which it tracks. Once driven against the femur it fractures, often transversely, right across the middle. These fractures commonly displace and usually require surgical repair. This involves using wires or screws or combinations of these to hold the patella together so that it can be moved a little while it's healing. Like the hand and elbow, the knee does not take kindly to prolonged immobilization. Held still, the knee will stiffen rather quickly. Once frozen, it may not thaw, so we go to some lengths to move the injured knee whenever we can. With well-fixed patellar fractures, we begin some motion in

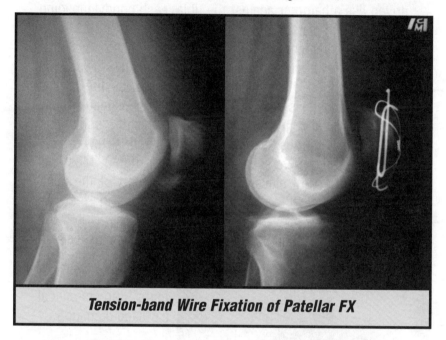

Tension-band Wire Fixation of Patellar FX

the first few weeks, and then slowly increase the motion with therapy and bracing. These injuries can easily take 6 months to recover and, since this is a fracture into the joint, there is always the possibility that, over time, osteoarthritis might set in.

The other common type of fracture that we see around the knee in the boomer age group is the tibial plateau fracture. The upper end of the tibia has two flares that accept the corresponding swellings at the lower end of the femur. These two flares are called the "tibial plateaus" (medial and lateral).

Articulating with each plateau is a corresponding swelling on the end of the femur called the femoral condyle (medial or lateral). One condyle meets up with one plateau. When the whole lower extremity is loaded from the bottom (the foot) up toward the hip, sometimes the joint in the middle gives first. When the knee is locked in full extension, the femur is driven like a hammer against the tibia, each condyle loading its underlying plateau. If the knee buckles toward the knock-knee, the lateral femoral condyle will be driven into the lateral tibial plateau, fracturing it. If the knee buckles toward the bowleg position, the medial side fractures, as the medial femoral condyle is driven into the medial plateau. These fractures usually involve falls from a height, snow and water-skiing injuries, vehicular trauma and a few rowdy athletic pursuits (I've seen a couple from rugby). Most will require surgery to elevate the depressed part of the joint.

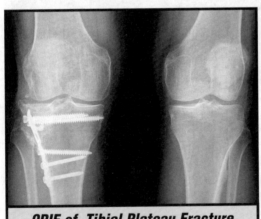

ORIF of Tibial Plateau Fracture with Plate and Screws

Some can just be braced and rehabilitated. Many are associated with other knee injuries including knee ligament tears and meniscal cartilage damage.

Just this last week I saw the CEO of a large aeronautics firm. As I was going through his orthopedic checklist, I noticed that he had all the usual boomer plus fighter jock maladies. He had dislocated his shoulder a time or two, starting with the Air Force Academy; now it was just a little stiff. He had some chronic low back pain after years in ejector seats and little or no trunk maintenance. Finally, he had recently had a tibial plateau fracture, sustained while snow skiing. He'd had it fixed by a surgeon back home with a beautiful result. He showed me the scar, and we both "ooohed" and "aaahed." His range of motion was essentially normal and he had no pain. The x-rays showed a skillful bit of carpentry with the titanium plate and screws in just the right place. I mentioned that if I had done this operation, I'd be out there showing it off.

In spite of the fact that his doc had done a beautiful job, I could see the subtlest irregularities that are inevitable in any restoration of this type. I choose the word "restoration" carefully, because this is much like gluing together a cracked porcelain vase. You may get it looking like a vase, it may even hold flowers again, but you'll always see the cracks and feel the glue lines where the cracks were. Once the smooth articular surface is damaged, that damage is permanent. You can't put Humpty Dumpty back together again. You can lift it up and mosaic it back together. It will do much better than if you hadn't done that, but it will never be a normal joint. Arthritis is likely to set in over time.

Arthritis sounds like a good place to close. Old Arthur is sort of the Grand Inquisitor for the knee. No matter what your offense, you will have to come before his court sometime. Arthur makes Judge Judy look like a chump. He even humbles Supreme Court justices, and he gives no mercy in his court. No good twist goes unpunished. Sure, your surgeon "just removed some cartilage from my knee," but did you ever think that maybe that cartilage was there *for a reason*?

Chapter 11: Foot and Ankle

When it comes to the problems of the foot and ankle it must be said that boomer women are victims of fashion, if only slightly less so than their mothers. Many cultures have strange rituals associated with keeping women "in their place" by attacking their feet. The most famous and extreme of these is the ancient Chinese custom of foot binding. In this demonic fashion, little girls' feet were bound and wrapped so tightly that the perfect adult outcome was a foot no bigger than a few inches in length, with the toes drawn up under the arch. Considering that this only died out late in the 19th century, one could hardly call this practice ancient.

The Western equivalent, high-heeled shoes, is not only persistent in our culture, but every time I think a rational wind is finally blowing the sails of this year's fashion, along hobbles some woman wearing high-heeled, platform-soled combat boots. She's lurching along on something I wouldn't prescribe as a joke, all in the name of being fashionable. For the life of me I don't understand why women would put up with wearing what I would call a prosthesis as opposed to a shoe: a five-inch heel, a narrow toe box, the forefoot all cramped into a point, sliding into a steep descent from this precarious perch. Worse yet, I can't for the life of me understand why I find it so damn sexy, but like any other healthy male, I do. And that, of course, is why these fashions persist.

Tomes have been written about this phenomenon. Psychologists have written of the accentuation of all the female erotic features, the lengthening of the legs, the perking up of the butt. Regardless of the whys and wherefores, you can count on this phenomenon persisting. I used to laugh at my wife Kathy and scold her about her footwear, blithely describing all the determinants of a "reasonable" woman's shoe. Then I finally went with her to shop for such a shoe and, guess what? They must be right there next to the unicorns, because I could never find one. At least I could never find one that was the least bit attractive or would go any better with a woman's workaday dress or suit than, say, wearing a mackerel for a tie would go with an Armani blazer.

So as an orthopedist, here's my rule. You can wear any damn shoe you like (and that goes for men who persist in wearing the male counterpart: the cowboy boot), as long you don't come to my office complaining about your feet. I am only going to tell you it's easier to fit the shoe to the foot than it is to fit the foot to the shoe.

The constellation of foot grievances related to female fashion includes bunions, hammer-toes, bunionette (little bunion on the little toe), metatarsalgia ("The balls of my feet hurt because I'm walking around in these damn high heels and that's where all the weight is going") and so on. In the early stages, all of these conditions are remedied by simply giving the foot some breathing room and letting it function like, well, like the foot is supposed to function. These are not complaints you see in cultures that don't wear shoes. You see women in India walking with bare feet, calloused to the thickness of the shoes we wear.

To illustrate the point that many foot problems are caused by fashion, the orthopedist or podiatrist will often have the patient stand on a piece of paper, then trace the outline of the foot with a pencil. Then he'll grab the patient's shoe and superimpose it over this tracing. Inevitably, the foot tracing swallows the shoe like some fat cat would a songbird, and one can see the tracing of the real foot longing for its freedom, hanging luxuriously over the edges of its prison.

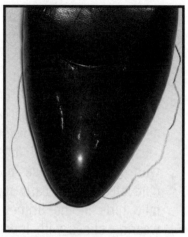

Most women strike some compromise and wear fashionable shoes for brief, fashionable occasions, knowing they will pay a short-term price. Then they find some reasonably nice-looking flat or shorter-heeled shoe to wear at work. They may even wear sneakers to and from work—something you can see on any street corner in Chicago or New York. This is one place where the new, more casually attired workplace of the dot-com culture is light years ahead of the boomers. But those Gen-X girls probably have a little closet full of high heels somewhere that they maybe just wear behind closed doors and after hours to turn on their twenty-something millionaires. No hard feelings, but don't expect high heels to disappear if the NASDAQ soars again.

Let's get specific about some of the most common foot complaints we see in boomers.

Bunions

A bunion is that painful prominence where the big toe meets the first metatarsal. For most people there is a slight bend away from straight at this joint, that is, the toe goes slightly away from the midline.

There is some significant genetic variability since some people, particularly some women, are born with a bit more of an angle here. This tendency can then be aggravated by the application of pointy-toed shoes and high heels. The great toe can be trained, corseted over ever farther away from the inside arch of the foot, until it bares the head of the metatarsal and the toe is almost completely dislocated from it. This takes time and determination but, with practice, these bunions can be cultivated by the early teen years. I see little girls in the Britney Spears crowd wearing shoes with four-inch heels and little razor sharp toes. These are painful feet in training.

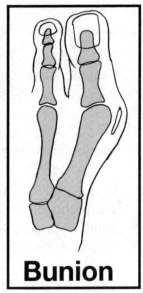

Bunion

From the first meeting between the boomer woman and her friendly neighborhood orthopedic surgeon, she and her doctor will be immediately at odds. She wants what he can't provide and he has a remedy that she probably won't accept—at least usually not at first. She wants a slim little foot that slips graciously and painlessly into any stylish shoe, no matter how diabolical the design. She's willing, almost anxious, to have surgery to meet this worthy goal. She doesn't want to be off her feet or out of work. One of those lunch-surgery jobs would be nice. Can you show me something with Laser? Her goals are simple, concrete, and easily and quite effectively communicated to the doctor, thank you very much. Then the communication starts to break down.

The doctor examines her foot. She does have a pretty good-sized bunion, and there are signs of chronic pressure and irritation over the bump. She has a big toe going off at a forty-five-degree angle, threatening to "under-lap" its neighbor, the second toe, seen currently running for its life by clawing up and out of the way into a hammertoe. Her foot is exceptionally wide from the spreading of the forefoot that routinely occurs with aging. (There it is again. You see, this whole boomer thing is *about aging*.) She's wearing a size shoe that would have fit well when she was a teenager. But though the size has been frozen in time, with time's cruel passage the foot has spread and twisted. This is a phenomenon almost unique to foot sizing. Though they accept a gradual inflation of belt sizes, people somehow assume that if they're a 6A at age eighteen, then they will forever be a 6A. Unfortunately, it doesn't work that way at all. The foot spreads and lengthens a little as the arches collapse and the youthful connective tissues, succumb to the chronic effects of applied gravitational theory. I see women who are wearing a shoe that is a full two sizes too small. Your classic "pound and half of potatoes in a one pound sack."

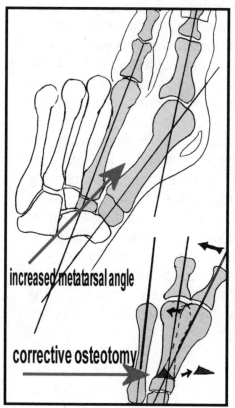

increased metatarsal angle

corrective osteotomy

Her x-rays reveal an even more serious problem. One big contributor to the tendency for the big toe's getting pushed over into a bunion deformity is a wider angle between the first and second metatarsals. Here's how this works.

Most people have less than 10 degrees of angle between the first and second metatarsals. If this angle is greater than, say, 20 degrees, then the great toe is even more at risk for getting pushed over when someone insists upon wearing constricting shoes. For our patient, this has surgical implications. You can't correct her deformity, by just lopping off the bump and straightening out the toe. In the lesser cases without this extreme metatarsal angle, the bump can be removed and the toe straightened without a prolonged recovery. If, as in our patient's case, the deviation is greater, then the metatarsal itself must be straightened to get rid of the deformity. This cutting through the bone, correcting the angulation and asking the toe to heal in a new position is called a "metatarsal osteotomy." Most of the time, if a person has significant bunion deformities, it takes one of these to straighten out her foot. Here's where the hopes of the patient and the goals of the surgeon begin to part paths.

How do you give her the bad news? You give it to her straight. With as little jargon and as much compassion as possible, the surgeon tries to explain that what we're looking at here is a pretty crooked foot and not just a painful bump. In order to fix this thing, it's going to take an operation that takes over an hour. This procedure involves cutting through the first metatarsal bone, rearranging its angle, pinning or screwing it into place, then trimming off the bump, realigning the toe and holding it all with either a cast or a clunky boot for at least six weeks. Can we do them both at the same time? You wouldn't want me to. The end results of these reconstructive procedures are generally good, but some of the most disappointed patients are those who come in thinking they are going to have what amounts to a cosmetic procedure, only to leave with pins, screws and six weeks in a cast. This is just another place where the patient and the surgeon should be very careful to make sure that they are both on the same wavelength.

Hammertoes, Metatarsalgia and Morton's Neuroma

Bunion deformity affects the great toe, but the lesser toes—the second through the fifth toe—are also a great source of discomfort and deformity. Like bunions, these lesser toe conditions are the direct consequence of constrictive shoe wear. You will never see any of these problems in cultures that don't wear shoes either. You may see the deformity we call *hammertoes*, but it won't be symptomatic. These conditions are the side effect of chronic constriction of the lesser toes by a too small toe box. The toe shortens, rears up like a spooked stallion and stays up there with the first joint of each toe, becoming its most prominent feature.

Projecting as it does above the plane of the rest of the toes, it takes the first impact from the roof of the toe box. This force is transmitted down along the shaft

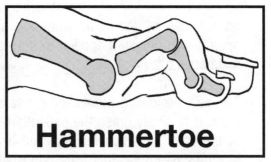

Hammertoe

of the toe, causing a direct transmission of this force down from the top of the foot to the sole or bottom. The toe comes crashing down on the metatarsal head, causing it to be more prominent. Pain under this metatarsal head is called *metatarsalgia*. These two conditions go hand in hand. Commonly, either the crooked toe or the prominent metatarsal head takes center stage, but both actors are in the same troupe.

Their fellow Thespian, *Morton's Neuroma*, becomes the headliner when the metatarsal heads get banged so tightly together that the nerves that run between them get pinched

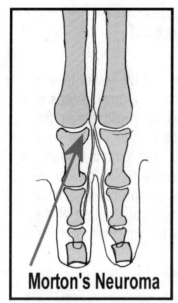

Morton's Neuroma

and beaten up. A neuroma, is a scarred up nerve, in this case, one that lives between two bones that won't stop banging heads.

This is most common in women, but is definitely seen in men, often related to cowboy boots or similar fashions with a bit of a heel forcing the foot to descend into a pointed shoe toe box. Morton's neuroma presents as pain in the metatarsal region and must be discriminated from garden variety metatarsalgia. The latter hurts right over the bones on the ball of the foot, whereas the neuroma hurts in response to pressure applied to the soft spots between the metatarsal heads.

The pain-provoking maneuver we save for last during this exam is to firmly grasp the patients metatarsals in the palm of the hand and then squeeze the heads together. In true Morton's neuroma, this little handshake elicits at the very least a startle response, and on occasion, the patient will exclaim, "Damn! I'm not paying you to hurt me!"

All these conditions at first respond to shoe modifications that give the poor banged up toes a little room to breath. Inserts can be prescribed and fitted into the shoe to relieve excessive pressure on this or that metatarsal head. Even in Morton's neuroma, patients often get relief with simple shoe modifications, inserts and awareness of the aggravating factors. When the conservative measures are unsuccessful, surgery to fix the hammertoes will correct both the problem in the toes and usually in the adjacent metatarsal heads that have been made prominent because of the hammertoes. There are many different ways of accomplishing this hammertoe correction. In fact, if you browse through a textbook on surgery of the foot and come to the page on hammertoes, you'll see at least ten different ways of doing this. The same is true for bunions; there are lots of different surgical approaches to the same problem. Herein lies another surgical truism: "Whenever there is more than one way of doing something, it usually means that there is no *one best way.*" This simply means that all of these operations work some of the time, in some surgeon's hands. For this reason, you need to ask your surgeon why he chooses to do the operation he's recommending to you. If his answer is, "The way I was doing it the last few months just wasn't working out, so I've switched to this new method," keep shopping.

The surgical procedure to correct Morton's neuroma is a bit more predictable. The only problem here is making sure the diagnosis is correct. This is a diagnosis based mostly on history and physical exam; there is no slam-dunk test, but the surgeon may wish to try an injection of lidocaine and cortisone in the suspected spot to see if the pain goes away temporarily. This is rarely effective as a long-term treatment, but it can be helpful in establishing the diagnosis in selected cases. The definitive surgery involves cutting out the damaged nerve. This, of course, leaves the patient with a numb patch on the inner side of the toe to which that nerve used to go. Patients are rarely aware of or bothered by this lack of sensation. Here again, we see how the Brain shows favoritism for the hand. The Brain would never tolerate this flagrant ablation of sensation in the hand. Outrageous! But the foot? Who cares? Can it still walk? OK? Well, that's all it's good for anyway…

That's the way we treat our feet in general. We don't treat

them at all unless they are injured or abused. Otherwise, we prefer to ignore them. One of my professors used to say, "Be kind to your feet; they outnumber people almost two to one." There's some wisdom in that.

Sprained Ankles

This is one of those common injuries that has a reputation for being more of a nuisance than a really serious injury. Ankle sprains get no respect. Everybody has sprained his or her ankle and it's always healed, right? Well, wrong, actually. A sprain is an injury to a ligament, and an ankle sprain is a tear in those ligaments that hold tight rein on a really tightly reined joint. The usual mechanism of injury is piddly enough. You're usually walking along minding your own business when you misjudge a curb, or maybe it's those bifocals again. That bottom part of the glasses, the real close-up part, is just great when you're reading, but when you're walking, it's all blurry right where your feet are supposed to be. And WHAM! Suddenly you invert your ankle. There's a sickening "pop" or whatever tearing collagen sounds like. Another case of "ascending numeritis": your number just came up. You have just changed your life for the next six to eight weeks. As the outside of your ankle starts to swell, you reach in your pocket for your Palm Pilot and tap out a message to the office: "Wounded in the French Quarter. Send cab to the House of Blues!" Then you check your calendar for the next month and a half, because things have just changed, walking-wise.

Like knee sprains, these come in three flavors: mild, moderate and severe. It's those mild and moderate ones that you're thinking about when you think they all do well. When you get into the complete tears—the severe sprains—you have a very painful swollen joint with some instability. This is

244

not a minor injury, and if there's any denial, it will remind the owner with every other step. There is often a good deal of swelling. I've heard some real Paul Bunyan descriptions— swelling of epic dimensions. "It swelled up like a basketball, doc!" "It was as big as a watermelon! I'm not kidding!" Let's just say, these swell some, OK? Swelling is bleeding from the ruptured ends of the ligament, and is almost always worst on the lateral or outside of the ankle. Swelling forces the foot down and into inversion, a precarious posture for walking. I guess that people who hobble around on these for a while are hoping against hope that this sprain will miraculously heal like the one they had in high school gym class. No way. Those days are over.

The first treatment principle in the management of adult ankle sprains is making sure that is *all* you are treating. If it's just a sprain, fine, but that has got to be another "diagnosis of exclusion." First, we have to make sure it isn't broken or something else isn't injured, like the Achilles tendon. This may seem easy, but it is, in fact, a common mode of mistreatment to overlook associated injuries in the face of what appears to be a simple sprain. I have a short checklist I give my residents, called "ankle sprains that aren't." This list includes several fractures that can go unrecognized, and the rupture of the Achilles and other tendons. Some times a "bad sprain" just isn't getting better because it is not a sprain at all, but a fracture of the anterior process of the calcaneus, or of the lateral process of the talus.

Once the diagnosis of sprain is confirmed by a negative x-ray exam and a good physical exam, the treatment is directed toward getting the swelling down, and getting the foot up into a neutral, walkable, "plantargrade[14]" position. This lets the ligament heal in the right position. Some patients have so much pain that they may need casting and may not be able

14 Plantargrade = the foot meeting the ground at a right angle to the leg; the position for walking.

to put any weight on the ankle at first. The goal should be to get the swelling and pain under control, get the foot up into a position where it can resume its weight-bearing role, and then initiate walking as soon as possible. Often patients with severe ankle sprains will require a brief period of splinting or casting while the swelling passes. We often use these removable walking boots, but removable is a double-edged sword. They are so convenient that they are sometimes conveniently removed as soon as the patient is out of the doctor's sight.

Once the swelling and pain are down and the foot is taking full walking duties, we usually apply a so-called ankle stirrup. These braces support the ankle, control the swelling and limit the motion in the wrong directions, without completely impeding ankle motion. These devices fit in a lace–up shoe and are usually worn for several weeks. I encourage those with the worst sprains to wear them for four to six weeks, though they rarely do. The hardest cases to treat are the most painful ones that get off on the wrong foot. Sometimes patients are first seen in the ER and given an ace-wrap, some ice and a pat on the back. Maybe crutches. After a few days, the foot is so swollen and inverted that it can't be brought up to the neutral, plantargrade position. In these cases you have to put on first one splint in the best position you can get that day, then slowly change the splints every couple of days until the foot comes up. Then you can slap it into a cast and get the patient walking on it. Walking is critical.

Once in the 1980s, Kathy and I were visiting a Mayo Clinic orthopedic classmate of mine at his beautiful home in Houston. He'd only lived there a short while and the first time Kathy and I walked in, our eyes were immediately drawn upward to the huge ceiling of the great room. Unfortunately, just a few feet inside the awe-inspiring entrance to his home was a single small step-off—very subtle, this little step. As we walked in, I saw Kathy suddenly drop off my radar screen to my left. She had completely missed the step and gone down in a heap with a badly sprained ankle. It literally began swelling before our eyes. But not to worry, she had fallen among two orthopedic surgeons and an orthopedic nurse. This was going to be the most immediately, thoroughly, expertly treated ankle sprain in history.

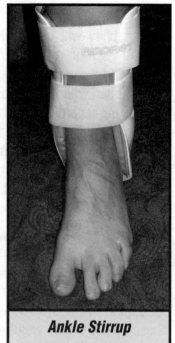

Ankle Stirrup

Margie ran and got the ice and wrapped the ankle with an ace wrap. Glenn and I got in his car and sped off to his office for tape and an air-stirrup. When we got back Kathy's ankle was elevated, iced, and wrapped and she was medicated and consoled. I used a technique of immediate taping, similar to what is used on professional athletes. We got an x-ray after we got back to San Antonio to confirm that nothing was broken. We made her get up and walk on it, and the swelling went down faster than we usually see, probably because it was so promptly treated. I taped and re-taped it for a week and then applied the air-stirrup. She wore that about two more weeks and by then had neither pain nor swelling. She had sustained a third degree (severe) ankle sprain and yet was back in action almost immediately and suffered no residual looseness or pain.

A few patients treated perfectly well may still develop residual instability of the ankle. It may become unpredictable and prone to acts of sabotage. The patient with chronic ankle instability will usually have an ill-defined mix of pain and laxity symptoms. We may have to do an x-ray stress test, which involves pulling on the ankle while taking an x-ray, to establish where it is loose. Minor degrees of ankle instability can be accommodated for by some sophisticated physical therapy balance training, but most significant instabilities will eventually involve surgical correction. Here the operation involves tightening up the lax ligaments. This is a common operation with predictably good results, but, as always, there is a several-month recovery period, and the first month is usually spent in a cast.

Fractures

The whole subject of ankle fractures consumes at least fifty pages in most textbooks of fracture treatment. I can summarize that wealth of information into a not-so-short sentence. There are lots of ways to break the ankle, but the tolerances for error are low and the stakes are high enough that many ankle fractures have to be fixed surgically. Remember that with the sloppy joints such as the shoulder you can tolerate some angulation and some rotation from a fracture. But with a tightly constrained joint like the

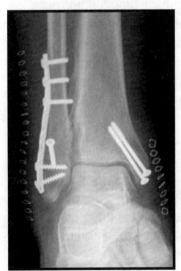

ankle, a millimeter either way can make a big difference. There are some minimally displaced fractures that don't screw up the alignment of the joint, and these can be treated with casting.

A lot of the more serious fractures involve the two prominences that are the ends of the tibia and fibula. Called the malleoli, these bumps are the stage doors of the ankle. Exit

248

stage left, you fracture the medial malleolus, exit stage right, and you've fractured your lateral malleolus. Worse yet, these malleoli can be injured together in a pattern we call a "bimalleolar" fracture.

In this case the fracture actually exits stage left and then re-enters stage right. Either way, the ankle is "bad busted," as they used to say in Texas, and it deserves an operation to fix it. These open reduction internal fixations usually involve a plate and screws on the skinny bone on the outside (the lateral malleolus), and a screw or two through the other (medial) malleolus. This is followed by a period of non-weight-bearing, usually around a month to six weeks. Then there follows another period of rehab, gait-training and strengthening. People who walk a lot in their jobs will be slowed down for several months. Limping and swelling can go on for at least a year, before leveling out. Though most people do well after ankle fracture surgery, many others go on to osteoarthritis.

Fractures of the 5ᵗʰ Metatarsal

Sometimes, nearly the same injury that can sprain or even break the ankle—the twisting, inversion injury—can do its damage a little lower down in the foot. It can fracture the base of the fifth metatarsal. This is sometimes mistaken for an ankle sprain and it is in that list of "ankle sprains that aren't" that I mentioned earlier. The swelling is on the same side as an ankle sprain and the mechanism of injury sounds the same. The tenderness will be a little lower down and directly over the fractured bone, but after a night of knife-and-gun-club trauma and a few cardiac arrests, you can forgive the harried ER doc for missing this one. And since the treatment isn't that much different from an ankle sprain, usually little harm is done.

We treat this injury with casting most of the time and sometimes just a hard-soled shoe, like the ones we put on patients after foot surgery. There is a variant of this fracture that occurs just a little farther down the bone towards the toes. If your surgeon seems a little more frantic, is talking about six weeks of non-weight-bearing, and maybe a screw being necessary if it doesn't heal, then you probably have this variant. Though fractures of the fifth metatarsal are usually pretty good actors, this small subset heals slowly and sometimes does require surgery.

Heel Pain

You can get pain in all sorts of places and for all sorts of reasons around the heel. I'll speak first about those conditions that relate to shoe wear, then discuss the very common condition of pain on the plantar surface of the heel, so-called "plantar fasciitis."

Some people are knobbier than others, particularly around the heel. If you are one of those poor unfortunates born with a knobby heel, you may get what's sometimes called a "pump bump," another painful bursitis. This one comes from direct irritation of the tissues between the heel bone and the back of the shoe. The bigger the bump, the more it continues to *get* bumped. The more its gets bumped, the bigger the pump bump will get. The treatment, of course, is to remove the source of the irritation by modifying your shoe wear until it calms down. Some athletic shoes have a little notch in the counter for the Achilles tendon. This usually takes the pressure off the pump bump for a while. Some people need surgery for this, but it's better to operate on the shoe than on the foot.

The more common pain in the heel is on the business side,

where the "rubber meets the road" on the plantar surface of the heel. Here there is an attachment of the strong ligament that spans the arch of the foot. This ligament is called the "plantar fascia" and its anchor on the heel bone is a firm one. It has to be; it 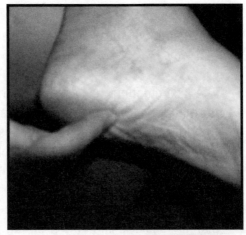 supports body weight with every step of every day forever. Sometimes that attachment gets overworked and painful. This is often associated with one or more of the following: a female patient, an overweight patient, or a patient with tight heel cords. You see this in skinny male joggers too, so don't get too glib, guys. I had this myself once and I'm neither female, nor overweight, nor tight of heel cord. But, for our example I'll choose an overweight woman in high-heeled shoes with heel pain.

She describes the pain as being on the underside of the heel. It is so localized that she can point to it with one finger. It hurts all day with every step, but it is at its absolutely hair-peeling worst when she first gets up in the morning. She can barely waddle into the john. She's tried various anti-inflammatories, all with little effect. She was told she might have a "heel spur." Unfortunately, her doctor got the x-ray report that showed she had a heel spur and sent her to the surgeon to have it removed. I say "unfortunately" because there is no correlation between the size, or even the presence, of heel spurs on an x-ray and heel pain. We see big spurs and no pain and big pain and no spurs. But often the primary care doctor will get the report of the heel spur and the patient will come to the surgeon convinced that removal of the spur will mean removal of the pain. It just doesn't work that way.

The examination reveals a rather anxious but otherwise normal appearing foot. All the toes are there and mostly in the right places. There is no stiffness and the skin looks OK. Where did you say it hurt? Right there? HERE? (Firm pressure from the examiner's thumb.) Ouch!

This kind of localized pain at the heel bone attachment of the plantar fascia is thought to be an injury, usually a chronic injury to this anchorage. These patients often have tight heel cords. As this patient so aptly demonstrates, walking around for a lifetime in high-heeled shoes will do this nicely. It will leave the patient uncomfortable when barefoot or in flats, but comfy enough when hanging ten over a pair of three-inch heels.

The calf muscle and the plantar fascia work together as one big spring. This spring starts up above the knee with the upper attachment of the calf muscle and attaches to the mobile fulcrum of the heel bone. When the calf muscle pulls through the heel bone, this force is transmitted through the ligaments of the plantar side of the foot, bringing the foot down toward contact with terra firma. The shock of contact is absorbed reciprocally up through the foot, across the heel bone and up to the calf muscles, which transmits it on up the chain of command. People with tight heel cords place more stress

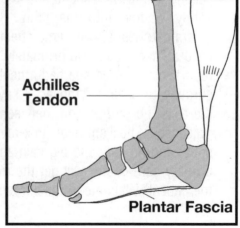

Achilles Tendon

Plantar Fascia

on this whole arrangement. It turns out that the weakest link in the chain is that place on the undersurface of the heel where the plantar fascia originates. When that area gets torn and beat up, the condition is called "plantar fasciitis," implying that there is inflammation of the injured fascia. There is, but the underlying cause is repeated injury, the inflammation is secondary.

The treatment is to reverse the heel cord tightness with selected stretching exercises. We also have prescription heel cups that fit in the shoe, cushioning the impact on the heel, and we have the dreaded "heel cortisone shot." Notice I haven't said this about any of the other shots I've prescribed. No shot feels great, but most of the others that I administer are not that bad for most patients. This one—plugging a needle into the heel—now that is serious pain. You can't really "freeze it." You just have to take your licks and let somebody plug your heel with this needle and a medicine that itself burns a little going in. I've seen grown men cry, and once I was cursed by a nun for giving her this shot. I'm not kidding. There I was, slipping my needle into Sister Mary Whatever's heel, and she let out this blood curdling F-word as if God would surely forgive her, if not me. Needless to say, I have great respect for this shot. I try everything else first. If somebody tells me they're ready to have "the shot," I have a video about the French Revolution that I make them watch.

Patients who don't get better with stretching, weight-loss, heel cups and the occasional shot, may need to be immobilized in a cast for a trial period of time. If all this fails, selected patients will respond to a surgical release of the plantar fascia. Plantar fascia release works by lengthening the ligament so that after it heals, there is less stress on its origin at the heel bone. Some doctors advocate doing this endoscopically through smaller incisions. I think the jury's still out on this one, and there has been some "over-promotion" of this procedure. Some doctors make it sound as if it is one of these "lunchtime" procedures. Get your fascia snipped over the lunch hour, go dancing at eight! In my opinion, most people should try months of conservative management without relief before they consider surgery. Then they should be prepared for a two- to three-month recovery period.

Achilles Tendon Rupture

They don't call this one "a career ending injury" for nothing. One minute Mark is back-peddling, trying to get some separation from that defensive line that's charging him. Let the receiver uncover, there he is! Plant the back foot and— SNAAAPP! "I'm going down, and I don't think I'll be getting back up. This time it's serious." Mark is thinking, "Here comes the John Deer," but then it occurs to him that this is only a weekend, flag football game! Hey! You're not supposed to have a career ending injury at an office party! What's the deal?

That snap, my friends, was the last gasp of Brave Achilles, strongman of the Greeks. Brave Achilles, who has for so long given so much and asked so little. Brave Achilles, who until as recently as the third quarter was able to run, jump, cut and bounce all over any time he damned well pleased. Brave Achilles, slain in his youth. You heard him shout as he died and you knew it was his last breath. He cannot be brought back, but will be carried off the battlefield, borne upon his own shield. We will never see the likes of him again. Mourn our fallen. Brave Achilles lies slain!

A little dramatic? Ask Vinnie Testaverde or Dan Marino or any other professional athlete who's had this happen to him and he'd say, "Yeah, that is a little dramatic. Hell, I never could spell 'Achilles' so I got to just callin' it my 'heel cord.' Just easier to spell; see what I mean?"

This is the largest tendon in the body. It is thick and strong and it is durable. But it is also attached to a very strong muscle group, which means that it can suddenly get jerked around. When someone suddenly chooses to advance while in the act of retreating, the single heel cord may be asked to sustain all the momentum of the body going hell-bent in one direction and then to turn that momentum on a dime and send it off hell-bent in the opposite direction. If we ask too much of this tendon, strong as it is, even it will fail. In fact, it will fail "catastrophically," as the engineers say. You don't just stretch this baby; you *blow* it. He *blew* or even *blew out* his Achilles, man. And that's exactly what they look like when you operate on them; as if something had exploded in there. The two ends of the torn tendon look like mop ends. The surgeon uses big strong sutures to patch Brave Achilles together, then entombs his remains in a fiberglass cast for up to six weeks. Then the wilted, stiffened leg and ankle start down the long road to never-quite-complete recovery.

This injury may also be treated without surgery. In this case one casts the foot down into a flexed position, so that the tendon ends are in the same general neighborhood. Gradually, over several weeks, the foot is brought back up. After at least six weeks of casting, another long run of therapy and recovery are ahead. The main reason to operate on these injuries is to attempt a little quicker recovery and perhaps have a tendon that is less likely to re-rupture. In either case it is unusual for someone with a complete rupture of the Achilles tendon to return to jumping sports at a competitive level. After going through and getting over this injury, most boomers are likely to modify their activities in a way that this is very unlikely to happen again.

So who among us hasn't sprained an ankle? Who hasn't come home and kicked those "dress" shoes off and padded around the apartment in her bare feet wondering why they don't let you do this at work? Who, reading this, doesn't know someone who has had a broken ankle, a bunion surgery, heel spurs or hammertoes? If you have nothing wrong with your wheels now, I'll bet you have at least once in your life—and the chances are very high that you will again. You can prevent some of these problems by wearing reasonable shoes, avoiding risky, competitive sports and looking out for dangerous steps, but many of the problems we see around the foot and ankle are simply the cumulative effect of bipedalism. If we hadn't gone from all fours to just walking on the hind limbs, the hands would be sharing some of the burden of locomotion. But believe me, the hands would never put up with high-heeled gloves.

Chapter 12: Fractures of the Long Bones

The orthopedic term of endearment for the big long bones of the arms and legs is "the Long Bones." There are three in each limb with one big one close to home and two smaller ones sharing the load distally. You've already met these players, but mostly at their joint ends. Now I'd like to discuss injuries to shafts of the humerus, the radius, the ulna, the femur, the tibia and the fibula. These bones of our upper and lower limbs have many similarities, and this derives from their having evolved from the limbs of our recent ancestors who walked on all fours. Yes, your hands were once lowly feet. They got their big break when the Brain decided to get this thing going bipedal. When they no longer had to assist the hind limbs in walking, the forelimbs became free to explore, evolve and poke around, and then to evolve some more. But deep within the core structure of this new fancy upper limb with its hand, there lies the remnant of the original walking design, like the three little taillights that tell you the car in front of you is a Mustang. When you see that big, long proximal bone and those two shorter ones beyond it, that means this limb had a former life as a leg. It used to be a weight-bearing limb, but it has been modified to serve the whims of the Brain, as acted out by the hand.

Since they are derived from weight-bearing bones, all the long bones have essentially the same structure. They are roughly circular in cross-section, long and tubular in the middle, and have complicated ends, usually participating in some important joint. The bone itself is arranged like a strong tube with a thick outer cortex and an almost complete absence of structural bone in the cavity created.

Fractures occur when the bone is stressed beyond its limits, usually by some violent act. Fractures can occur from collisions, vehicular and otherwise, sudden decelerations (falls, jumps and crashes), sudden twists, direct blows and you-name-it. Most boomers are a little too early for osteoporosis to be a common player, so most long bone fractures will occur from significant trauma. In midlife we usually walk away from ground height falls, as these are called with old folks. In other words, a boomer can

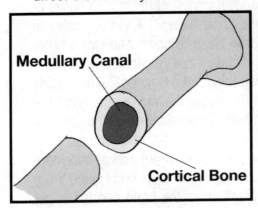

Medullary Canal

Cortical Bone

do a face plant, stand up, shake it off and walk away. This would almost never be the case in an elder person. You have to unexpectedly hurl a boomer at something going 60 miles an hour, or push him or her over the edge on the last run of the last day of that last lift ticket. I just saw a colleague who dumped his bike on the levee, not far from our hospital. There is three-inch rise of asphalt that drops off precipitously, on either side of the raised pathway. Put a guy in toe clips and let him accidentally slide over that edge and BAM! Doctor has an open, both-bone forearm fracture with a little bit of the radius left behind with the asphalt. This fellow is being skillfully treated by one of my partners, but he's got more rehab work ahead of him.

The absolute best mechanism of injury for the long bones, the "King of Them All" and the old standby when the ER seems slow, is the motorcycle. You just don't see a lot of orthopods riding motorcycles. You dump your Hog at even 30 miles per hour and, leather and helmet or no, you are in a world of hurt. One femur and two open "tib-fibs" are not uncommon. That's what we call a shattered leg with the bones sticking out through the skin and the jeans and the boots. An open tib-fib is an abbreviation for a "combined fracture of the tibia and fibula." We used to call open fractures "compound" fractures, but people confused it with "comminuted" which means broken into more than several pieces. People were always telling us they had a "compound" fracture when, in fact, it wasn't an open fracture at all, just one with a lot of pieces. Believe it or not, compared to open fractures, these are good news because true open fractures are a surgical emergency. They should be taken to the operating room and surgically washed out as soon as possible. If more than six hours of time has elapsed from the initial injury, the chance of permanent infection starts climbing. Most long bone fractures, open or closed, will be treated by surgical fixation. We will rod it, plate and screw it, externally fix it or in some other way stabilize it. You will not die of your broken bone, but you can die from the diseases of recumbence: pneumonia, blood clots, fat in the lungs from the shattered bones, infections of the urinary tract and so forth. If you break your femur, one tib-fib and a humerus, we'll fix them all, as soon as possible, so that we can get you out of bed. Bed Kills. Years ago doctors understood this, but our ability to get people up within a short period of time was limited. We placed people in traction for six weeks at a time. We cast severely broken legs that took three or four months to heal. A broken humerus hung limply in a sling waiting for spring to come. Then along came the Swiss.

Starting in the late 1950s, the Swiss began paying the same detailed attention to orthopedic fracture fixation they had previously focused on watch making and banking. They established an institute that began studying better ways of fixing broken bones. This group was called the

ArbeitsgemindsschaftOsteosynthesefragen, or "AO" for short. Beginning in the 1970's the techniques and hardware developed by this institute have gradually become the standard for fracture fixation. That's why you don't see kids hanging up in traction any more. We will rod that femur, plate that tibia or whatever else is necessary to get you up and going.

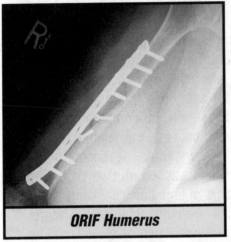

ORIF Humerus

In general, fractures of the biggest bones, the femur, the tibia and the humerus, do well with rods. These rods are placed through an incision over the end of the bone. First, a guide wire is passed inside the bone and across the fracture into the far end of the bone. This guide wire can act as a guide for reamers if one chooses to ream up to a certain rod size. Think of this reamer as bone "roto-rooter" that follows the guidewire, opening up the bone's inner canal for the rod to follow. The same guide wire will guide the rod into the canal and across the fracture, once the proper size and length have been selected. The reamings actually act as bone graft, because all these nice marrow cells get spread around the fracture sight. That's where bone cells come from: blood and marrow cells. Best of all, the fracture site itself is not even exposed. Everybody's happier when rods can be used. The fracture is usually instantly fixated and rendered rigid enough that the pain improves dramatically. We can get the patient out of bed.

Some fractures cannot be rodded safely. Fractures that extend toward the ends of the bone may not be amenable to rodding. Other fracture combinations may make rodding not the best strategy. In such cases plating the fracture with metal plates and screws is often the next choice. This is most commonly seen in fractures of the forearm bones, which we routinely plate. We also may plate the fibula while rodding

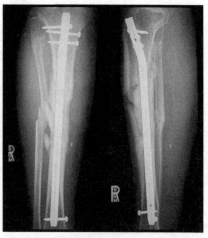

the adjacent tibia, so sometimes techniques are used in combination.

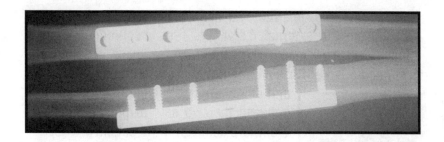

Once the bone is fixated, now the fun begins. Neighborhood joints do not take well to broken bones in their midst. They get cranky and stiff. Or they may suffer the indignation of being imprisoned in a cast, falsely convicted as an accessory to the crime of the fractured bone. Like the bone, the joint will be held without bond for six weeks, unable to do any of the things a respectable joint is supposed to do. When joints are immobilized, the muscles surrounding them get flabby. They go on vacation to the Caribbean and come back wasted so badly that when that cast finally comes off, you're thinking, "Whose leg is that?"

Another advantage of the modern fracture fixation

techniques is that we can move the joints right away, much of the time. We only use casts infrequently, such as after fracturing and plating both the radius and the ulna. Whenever we can, we try to fix all the broken limbs as surely and as quickly as possible. Then we try to get everything moving. Physical and occupational therapists usually begin treating these seriously injured patients in the hospital bed, soon after surgery. Even if the patient is lying in an Intensive Care Unit bed, there are the therapists, trying to move the broken limbs so they don't get stiff and so the patient doesn't get sick. Movement is the key not only to preventing joint stiffness but also blood clots, and other more serious medical complications like pneumonia.

There is another apparatus we use around fractures of the long bones: the external fixiter. We first encountered this concept when discussing fractures of the distal radius. I described a fixiter for such a wrist fracture, with pins above

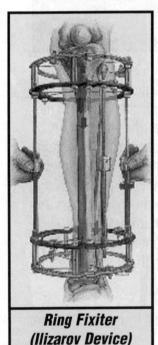

**Ring Fixiter
(Ilizarov Device)**

and below the fracture and a metal bar between the two sets of pins to keep them in place—as if the patient's wrist were in traction while he or she is walking around.

A somewhat more complicated arrangement allows for incredible variety in fixating some of the worst fractures, particularly in the leg. Lower extremity external fixiters tend to utilize combined techniques of half pins into the bone from one direction only and small wires that suspend bony fragments between iron rings around the limb. These so-called "hybrid" external fixiters may look gruesome, but they allow almost any fracture to be stabilized, no matter how much bone loss there has been and how much soft tissue damage. In fact, perhaps the biggest advantage of the external fixiters in certain open fractures is the access they allow to the damaged soft tissues. The surgeon can often leave the frame on while working to achieve soft tissue coverage.

Not all fractures heal. The more energy absorbed by the bone at the time of failure, the more soft-tissue stripping and the more the comminution, the more there is a chance that the fracture will fail to unite—what we doctors call "non-union." The non-union rate varies from bone to bone, but it's always in the single digits. By this I mean that if a hundred long bones break, we can expect, say, 95% of them to heal and 5% of them to go on to non-union. Fractures that are healing slowly, we may call a "delayed union," but the distinction is semantic. Some fractures just stall out and never finish healing. Some will respond to external electrical fields, such as pulsed electromagnetic fields. This Wizzard of Oz stuff actually works and heals a good percentage of long bones that don't heal the first time around. Fractures that are slow to heal and do not respond to electrical stimulation require an operation to stimulate healing at the fracture site, usually with bone grafting.

There are some new technologies on the horizon that are being developed to heal fractured bones. The most exciting of these techniques takes the actual chemicals and materials involved in bone healing and injects them into the fracture site. We now have purified "bone morphogenic protein" or BMP. This is a protein that changes the things around it into bone, or rather "induces" things around it to make bone. We can mix that with a little de-mineralized bone matrix, sprinkle in the BMP, maybe coax a few of the patient's own marrow cells out of early retirement, and there you have it. Healed!

Many bone-graftings may involve redoing the fixation, as well. This may mean changing from rod to plates, or to a different type of rodding.

In the end, most long bone fractures can be made to heal, though for a few unlucky individuals this is a prolonged ordeal. Most of the time, the limb regains most of its former function and the fracture incident fades into the forgotten past. The most likely conditions to linger are those in which the adjacent joints have been afflicted with arthritis during healing and recovery; and those in which weakness in the muscles has developed, meaning that the muscles will possibly never be restored to their former glory. Some people will have to live with some aching pain when the weather changes.

Doctors usually leave the internal hardware inside the patient. There has to be a pretty good reason to take out a two-foot long rod, such as irritation in an adjacent tendon or ligament. Mostly, we leave these things in so you'll have something to talk about at the cocktail party. "Did I tell you about skiing last year at Elk Park? Broke my tibia in three places. Yeah, the ski trip from Hell! Got a two-foot metal rod in there! Wanna see my X-ray?"

Chapter 13: Osteoporosis

This Is Not Just a Disease of Little Old Ladies

It used to be said, "You enter life through the birth canal and exit it through the femoral neck." In other words, one day you're born and then many years later you die when you break your hip. There is still a lot of truth in that statement and the events leading up to that fatal hip fracture are largely preventable. The prevention and treatment of osteoporosis begins right now, in women age 30 and up. And that is the main theme of this chapter. We're going to talk about the disease itself, its cause, its prevention and its treatment, but we should never lose sight of the fact that the problem we're talking about kills people, just a surely as a heart attack or cancer. After a century of advances in the treatment of hip fractures, the mortality rate at one year is still around 20%.

Over 25 million Americans—mostly women—develop symptomatic osteoporosis later in life, but the process begins much earlier. Osteoporosis is one of those diseases whose name describes the pathological process itself. Osteoporosis is actually "porous bone" or loss of the normal bone density and quality. Bone is a matrix with criss-crossed bone holding the structure together. With osteoporosis, the bone deteriorates into little islands that can collapse on themselves as the bone linkages fade away. The skeleton is one of the most complicated and misunderstood organs. It not only provides all the structural support for posture, locomotion and protection of all the "vital organs" but it also is the storehouse of crucial minerals, especially calcium, and the nursery for most of our blood cells. Though you may think of bone as an inert, wood-like scaffolding, it is in fact an incredibly dynamic, ever-changing plant that is sensitive to mechanical stresses, chemical and hormonal shifts in the rest of the body, diet and sickness. The level of calcium in the blood is one of the body's most closely regulated parameters and the brain will gladly borrow great stores of calcium from the bones to keep its other vital organs humming away. The bone is also a "use it or lose it" tissue, just like muscle. If the bone isn't stressed a little, it weakens. Though this is a huge worry for astronauts in weightless space flight, it is an even more practical problem for sedentary couch and mouse potatoes whose daily physical activity may not stimulate the skeleton enough to prevent gradual loss of bone mass.

Though osteoporosis occurs in both sexes, for all practical purposes this can be considered a disease of women. The men that get osteoporosis are usually those who have some disease that switches their metabolism to a more feminine chemistry or who are put to bed for more than two weeks for surgery or illness. The best example of this would be a 70 year-old man with prostate cancer who has had to undergo physical or chemical castration to treat the spread of his disease. Alcoholism, the resultant liver disease, smoking and cortisone can all do the same thing, but for this discussion, we can speak directly to midlife women. But even among women there are racial and genetic differences: osteoporosis is much more common in Caucasian and Asian women and less common in women of African ancestry. The disease results from a gradual loss of the quality and density of bone—as women age. However, the process begins much earlier in life than the fractures that herald clinical osteoporosis.

How and When the Damage Is Done
One in four women age 45 already have measurable

osteoporosis and 9 of 10 women over age 75 have measurable osteoporosis. What does this tell us? Two things: First, the events leading up to skeletal weakening must begin earlier in life than menopause and second, that whatever causes this disease must get worse with aging. Here's how it works. Osteoporosis can be thought of as a threshold of bone mass below which the bone can't do its job and it fails. That failure may be a broken hip, a broken wrist or a compression fracture of the spine, but in all cases, the skeleton has just gotten so weak and brittle that what might be an innocent fall for a teenager, becomes a life-threatening event. In other words, osteoporosis is a gradual downhill slide to some threshold where factures begin occurring. So, it matters greatly how high the hill was before the slide started and how steep the hill is once that slide has begun. For this reason, the best strategy for prevention is to maximize bone mineral density at its peak before age 26, and to slow down the rate of bone loss as much as possible after menopause.

For most women the sentinel event that starts the slide down the hill toward osteoporosis is menopause. Menopause is a gradual giving out of the ovaries, and the result is a dramatic decrease in the ovaries' main product, the female hormone estrogen. Since estrogen in intimately involved in maintaining bone mineral density in women, when it diminishes, the skeleton begins to weaken, unless the estrogen is replaced. But it is also critical just how solid the skeleton was at the onset of menopause. Some women have done everything right, and have raised their bone mineral densities to higher levels than others. Their bones are stronger from exercise and perhaps good genes. When these women hit menopause their bone mass has more mineral to spare, and even if they lose bone mass at the same rate as their weaker-boned sisters, they will not begin to suffer fractures for a much longer time. Conversely, some women have done all the wrong things prior to menopause. They have done nothing to boost or even protect their bone mineral densities and as soon as their ovaries fail, look out! Though they will start down that hill toward osteoporosis at the same rate, they will get there much sooner because they started closer to the level of bone loss at which fractures begin to occur.

From a purely historical accounting you could say that though women give calcium to men through breast-feeding their sons, men never return the favor. Childbirth and particularly breast-feeding place higher demands on women at a critical time, when they might otherwise be building their bone mass up for that later winter of their lives. The daily calcium requirement for a man at age 20 is 850 mg/day. But for a breast-feeding woman of the same age it is 2000 mg/day. If she isn't making up that difference, she's simply losing mineral in the bone bank and she'll be paying for it later.

How it all Works: Following Calcium from Your Broccoli to Your Bone

Calcium metabolism is a complex interaction of dietary intake, absorption of calcium through the gut, transport of that calcium to the cells that need it right now—like the beating heart—storage of the calcium that's needed for later and finally clearance through the kidneys of any excess calcium that isn't needed now or later. Many organs including the skin, the gut, the kidneys, the liver, the pituitary gland, the parathyroid glands, the ovaries in women, the testes in men, and finally the bones are involved in this intricate dance. Unfortunately, if anybody on this conference call doesn't do his job correctly, the result will usually be seen first in decreased strength of the bone. This is because the need for elemental calcium is so critical for so many other cells in the body, that the brain regulates this commodity very closely and isn't at all hesitant to make a withdrawal from the huge stores of calcium banked as structural mineral in the bone. The result is less bone mass and less bone strength.

The gut needs Vitamin D to absorb dietary calcium. Vitamin D comes from the skin when it is exposed to ultraviolet sunlight, and food (butter, eggs, food fortified with vitamin D such as milk and some breakfast cereal, and cod liver oil). Because most people do not get enough vitamin D from food and sunlight, a multivitamin may be the most consistent source of vitamin D. The recommended daily allowance is 400 I.U. Vitamin D then has to be modified, once in the liver and again in the kidney before it's actively able to facilitate calcium absorption in the gut. If there is adequate calcium available for absorption in the gut and adequate vitamin D to get the job done, then the brain has to decide where this calcium should go. Should it be sent immediately to the cells that need it, or do all the customers already have enough calcium for right now, in which case, can it be banked in the bones? If some is available for deposit in the bones, then the estrogen from the ovaries, growth hormone from the pituitary and thyroid hormone in normal levels are all necessary to pull that off. Finally, the bones have to be getting enough mechanical stimulus—they need to be gainfully employed against gravity and muscular resistance—to justify saving the available calcium. If any links in this chain are missing or misfiring, then the calcium that would otherwise be stored in bone just gets cleared out through the kidneys.

So let's look at what could go wrong, what could get between the calcium in your spinach and its storage in your bones. Obviously, there could be a low calcium intake in the diet. This is all too common in our modern diet. For instance, many women are lactose intolerant and therefore have had a lifetime of avoiding calcium-rich dairy products. Many diets are deficient in the leafy green vegetables like broccoli and kale that would provide an excellent source of calcium. So problem number one is usually too little calcium actually entering the pipeline.

Then there is the subtle interaction of calcium and its sister mineral phosphorus. Calcium and phosphorous are regulated by the same mechanisms and in a way compete for the attention of the gut when it comes to absorption and the kidneys when it comes to excretion. Diets high in phosphorous will inhibit absorption of calcium. Well, some of us are old enough to remember when you could go down to the drug store soda fountain and get a cherry phosphate. All carbonated soft drinks are high in phosphorous and the woman who drinks Diet Coke all day, thinking she is keeping her figure, is actually losing her bone instead. Carbonated soft drinks are the major offenders in the modern diet.

Nowadays we make exposure to the ultraviolet rays from the sun sound like the work of the Devil, but some sun exposure supplies crucial vitamin D by interacting with the skin. Most persons who live above the Mason-Dixon Line are vitamin D deficient in the winter unless they take a multi-vitamin daily. The liver and kidney convert vitamin D to the form that is active in the gut, and this process is less efficient with age. Some of the most osteoporotic women we have ever treated are the older pale blue-eyed Irish Catholic nuns who spent a life wearing the habit, and compounded their genetic predisposition for bone loss with an almost complete absence of vitamin D from the sun.

So if the calcium gets into the pipeline and then gets absorbed without incident, next it needs to get into the bones. Here we get into genetics. In fact, 85% of the risk for getting osteoporosis is genetically determined. If your mother had a hip fracture from osteoporosis, you are twice as likely as the average woman to have one yourself later in life. Some races just seem to do this better than others and the ones that don't do it at all well are the lighter skinned, pale-eyed folks. But for all women, the loss of estrogen after menopause makes it a lot harder for the calcium absorbed to find its way into the structure of the bone. This osteoporotic bone is structurally weaker than normal bone, because there is less bone substance to withstand the stresses imposed on the skeleton.

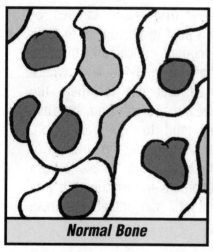

Normal Bone

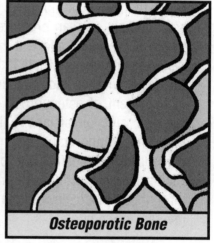

Osteoporotic Bone

In New Orleans we live in mortal fear of termites. We are blessed with many grand old homes and the unique buildings of the French Quarter, but they are all under attack by the fierce wood-eater, the Formosan Termite. Many of these gracious old mansions remind me of osteoporotic elderly women. They may look great from the outside but sometimes the walls and floors are eaten through to a honeycomb of cellulose, much like the thinned-out, fracture-prone bone of women with this disease.

In the end osteoporosis is a disease that results in fractures and the most commonly fractured bones are the hip, the spine, the wrist and the shoulder. Most of these fractures occur with a fall, but not always the kind of fall that might be expected to result in a break. A simple fall on the outstretched hand may cause a splintered wrist or a shattered arm. A woman may trip at home, fall to the floor and sustain a life-threatening hip fracture. So if that's what we're trying to avoid here, how can we do that?

What You Can Do to Help Yourself

Now that you understand the origin and causes of osteoporosis, we can organize a plan to prevent it, to slow the loss of bone before it becomes critical and even to restore bone mass when it has reached the level where fractures have already occurred. But this is where the management of osteoporosis becomes confusing, because patients and physicians alike tend to mix prevention, maintenance and actual treatment—that is, the *reversal* of osteoporosis—together into one big gumbo. I'd like to keep each separate, starting with prevention and working our way through to those newer treatments that actually promise reversal of the bone loss.

Prevention of Osteoporosis

When a woman barely eats and exercises to extremes, her menstrual periods cease and her estrogen level becomes the same as that of a much older, post-menopausal woman with osteoporotic bones. Repeated stresses on this abnormally weakened bone, results in a fatigue fracture or stress fracture, much like a coat hanger that is bent over and over again until it finally breaks.

The first step in the prevention of osteoporosis is the awareness that this condition begins whenever a woman starts making withdrawals from her calcium bone bank. This may even begin in her teens if she diets or exercises too much, or in her twenties after having and then nursing several children. It may begin with the genetic predisposition, and then be compounded by poor dietary habits, smoking, over- or under-exercise, cortisone treatments and lactose intolerance. Problems with any of the organs involved in the metabolism of calcium—skin, kidneys, liver, thyroid, parathyroid, gut, or pituitary—may severely aggravate the bone loss. But the critical step in prevention is recognizing that you are at risk if you have a family history, have the predisposing genetic pedigree, or have any of the above risk factors.

Bone mineral density is a test measuring whether a woman is trending toward osteoporosis and I recommend that any woman over 40, who is at risk for osteoporosis, have her bone mineral density measured. An ultrasound of the heel is a painless, low-cost screening test that takes 2 minutes but is not as accurate or reproducible as a nuclear hip and lumbar spine bone density test. The current gold standard is the DEXA or Dual Electron X-ray Absorbtiometry. This test can be used to measure bone density in the spine, wrist, or hip. It involves a tenth the radiation of a chest x-ray. The DEXA can also be used to follow changes in bone density with treatment. Repeat tests for comparison should be of the same bone. Two years is the soonest we could expect to see a meaningful change.

These bone mineral density tests are reported as deviations from a mean (average) expected bone density for your age (the Z score) or deviations from your peak bone mass at age 26 (the T score). If you are more than 2.5 "standard deviations" from either the T or Z score in any bone, you have significant osteoporosis and your fracture risk is high. The T score is considered the most significant. But any loss of bone mineral density as evidenced by a number less than that expected for your age, is a reason to change your habits and consider treatment. Bone density tests have been helpful tools for screening for osteoporosis but paradoxically, an improved bone density does not always correlate with a decrease in fractures. This may go back to the quality of bone (the cross-linked structure) but look for more research to explain this phenomena and more information on osteoporosis drugs *proving* that they prevent fracture.

Prevention of osteoporosis means avoiding those factors that deplete bone formation and encouraging those that enhance bone formation. You should avoid smoking, alcohol, carbonated phosphate containing beverages, caffeine in high doses, protein-rich or salty foods and inactivity. You should eat a diet high in calcium like dairy products, leafy green vegetables, beans and nuts, and whole-grain cereals. Even with admirable dietary habits, most women will fall short of the daily calcium and vitamin D intake necessary to maintain bone mass. Most physicians recommend taking a calcium supplement of 1000 mg/day until menopause and then 1500 mg/day after that. Citracal (calcium citrate) with vitamin D is among the best absorbed and does not require acid in the stomach to be absorbed. Five or six flavored regular Tums (calcium carbonate), each containing 200-300mg of calcium, are an inexpensive alternative and are best absorbed if taken with a meal.

With respect to calcium in the diet, as people age, many lose their ability to effectively absorb calcium and lactose, found in milk and milk products. They experience gastrointestinal discomfort when drinking up to four glasses of milk a day, which is the equivalent of the calcium supplements I recommend. A little milk in one's coffee or in a container of yogurt does not provide enough calcium. One cup of milk has 300 mg. of calcium, one ounce of cheese has 150-257 mg, and yogurt has 300-450 mg. per 8 ounces. Even though calcium is found in green leafy vegetables, it is unlikely that a person will be able to eat enough each day to supply the calcium that is needed. One would have to eat twelve servings of kale, boiled collard greens, or broccoli to get over 1000 mg. of calcium daily.

While calcium alone will not prevent osteoporosis, if you do not take it, you will get the disease earlier if you are so predisposed. People also require 400-850 IU/day of vitamin D. One multivitamin tablet usually contains 400 IU. No scientific evidence exists for the use of magnesium in skeletal health, though you wouldn't know that reading the lay literature.

Beyond avoiding the villains, adopting good dietary habits and taking calcium supplementation, a woman should get regular, reasonable exercise. Bone responds to weight bearing and resistance with a healthy increase in bone mass. It responds to overuse and unnatural stresses by fracturing. This is not some fine line that's hard to define. Persistent pain in the weight-bearing bones in response to high levels of exercise is a warning sign of an impending fracture. Reasonable exercise includes daily, non-impact aerobic activities like brisk walking, treadmill, cycling, swimming, and light weight or resistance training. The importance of regular exercise cannot be overemphasized in maintenance of skeletal health.

Calcium Needs of Women	
Children below age 10	850mg
Teenagers	1200-1500mg
Breast feeding mothers & pregnant women	2000mg
Before menopause	1000mg

After menopause
   If not taking estrogen
   If taking estrogen
	
	1500mg
	1000mg

Menopause and the Downhill Slide

So far we've discussed what a woman can do to climb as high as she can, up on that hill of bone mass before the eventual downhill slide begins. Now we will look at what she can do to keep from sliding down the hill abruptly after menopause and then what she can do to restore her bone if she has already slipped to below that threshold where the fractures of osteoporosis start occurring.

How abrupt is the fall? It is estimated that a woman can lose 1/3 of her bone mass in the first 6 years after menopause! So a woman who has a marginal bone mineral density at age 50 when her ovaries give out, can be at serious risk for fracture within a very short time. The mood changes, the hot flashes, the "drying out" of the mucous membranes, the thinning of the hair and all the other bothersome symptoms of menopause are more obvious and seem more in need of immediate attention, but in the end, it's the osteoporosis that can kill you.

For many years, physicians have recommended post-menopausal women take estrogen supplement and we know for certain that women who take estrogen after menopause protect themselves against bone loss. But there are several controversies about the use of estrogen. First, though we know that estrogen protects women's bones, it is less clear that it prevents fractures over time. I say less clear, because everyone just assumed that taking estrogen would be good, and therefore the rigorous scientific studies that would show that taking estrogen prevents fracture—the treatment endpoint in osteoporosis—are lacking. This is important because there is also a downside to estrogen replacement after menopause. Blood clots are slightly more likely, and if you take estrogen for more than five years after menopause, you have a slightly increased risk of breast cancer and uterine cancer. So what we have here is a classic risk/benefit trade-off. A woman whose mother died of breast cancer is just not going to want to take estrogen to prevent osteoporosis. She'll take her chances with the fractures and that's understandable. We can tell her that her risk of developing an osteoporosis-related fracture is as high as her *combined risk* for breast, uterine and ovarian cancer, but she still can't be expected to take estrogen. Here I think every woman has to sit down with her doctor and discuss her own personal pros and cons, based on family history, and her current bone mineral density as measured by DEXA or some other bone mineral density testing.

The controversy might be settled in the near future with the emergence of the new "designer estrogens", or "anti-estrogens" originally formulated as treatments for breast cancer metastases. Evista (raloxifene) is a new type of drug that is called a "Selective Estrogen Receptor Modulator" or SERM. The first of these drugs was tamoxifen, which is now widely used to slow the metastases from breast cancer. These drugs work by blocking estrogen receptors at the breast. But it was discovered that in doing so, a chemically similar medicine, raloxifene, also protected post-menopausal women against bone loss and it had none of estrogen's worrisome effects on the uterus or breast. So here may be a drug that works against bone loss, without increasing the risk of breast or uterine cancer. There are good studies showing this improvement in bone mass as measured by DEXA. Prevention of fractures will hopefully be scientifically confirmed in the future. The long-term side-effects are unknown since the drug has only been used a few years in humans. In the short-term, raloxifene is associated with a slight increase in blood clots and many patients discontinue it due to hot flashes.

Recently at least one long term study of so-called "hormone replacement therapy" or HRT concluded that women taking combinations of estrogen and progesterone were at higher than expected risk of heart attack, stroke and breast cancer. It is important to note these studies were in women taking two hormones. But the data from this and other studies make this whole area of discussion even more controversial.

What about calcium supplementation after menopause? Well, clearly it should continue, but many women think that just taking calcium alone is somehow going to prevent osteoporosis and fractures. It will not. The truth is that a woman who does not have an adequate daily dietary intake of calcium will be more at risk for fracture than one who does, but that calcium alone is not enough. It needs to be combined with vitamin D, exercise, avoidance of the things that deplete calcium, and probably SERM therapy for those women at higher risk of breast or uterine cancer. In established cases of osteoporosis, only therapies that restore bone mass—and calcium alone can't do that—will help decrease the rate of fracture.

What If You Already Have Osteoporosis?

The diagnosis of osteoporosis is made by bone mineral density test (DEXA scan etc.), looking at the thoracic spine on a routine lateral chest x-ray, or, all too commonly, by a fracture resulting from minimal trauma. Sometimes the fractures are microscopic and cause back and bone pain.

Don't assume that your doctor will proceed from the fracture toward a comprehensive evaluation and treatment plan for osteoporosis. This is particularly true for the orthopedic surgeon who may be called upon to fix your broken hip, or broken wrist. He's going to be occupied with the treatment of the fracture itself, and though he may recommend that you follow up with your internist or family doctor for treatment of the underlying cause of the fracture—your osteoporosis—it will probably be up to you to take that action.

Once the diagnosis is established, it means that you have slid down the hill of bone mass, to a point where fracture has either occurred or is likely. With prevention the idea was to get as high as possible on the bone mass hill before menopause. With bone maintenance after menopause, the idea was to stay up there on the hill and not slide too far down. Now the goal becomes both arresting the slide down the hill and if possible, climbing back up it to a level where fractures will be less likely to occur. All the strategies mentioned before still apply—take your calcium and vitamin D, get your exercise, etc.—but now we have to look for ways of restoring bone mineral density. Estrogen, SERMs or any drug that protects the bone against further bone loss is considered an "anti-resorptive" agent. Now we can add to that group, several drugs that don't just stop bone loss but restore it. Until quite recently this simply was not possible. Now we have agents that can actually increase bone mineral density and there is one treatment on the horizon that appears even more potent.

The agents which restore bone mass are called the "biphosphonates". These compounds work by inhibiting the natural resorption of bone that goes on as part of daily metabolism. Bone is constantly being laid down and resorbed throughout life. After menopause, the balance tips in the favor of resorption and destruction. These drugs tip it back in favor of bone formation. In doing so, they can actually restore bone mineral density in osteoporotic bone. Fosamax (alendronate) is commonly used. It can be given in a single weekly dose, which seems well tolerated with fewer gastrointestinal side-effects than daily Fosamax. Biphosphonates may be irritating to the esophagus, and so they have to be taken in the morning, flushed down with adequate water and followed by one hour of remaining upright and not eating. If taken at bedtime, for instance, esophagitis could be a problem. In addition to Fosamax, Actonel (risendronate) is available as a daily pill and should soon be approved for weekly use. The biphosphonates are more powerful than designer estrogens in building stronger bones and have been demonstrated to reduce vertebral fractures. We need more proof that they prevent hip fractures. Biphosphonates may only need to be taken for a few years because they remain in the bones for many years. Because of their very long-term stay in bone, we cannot fully predict the long-term effects, so doctors are hesitant to use these drugs in younger women with osteoporosis.

Miacalcin (calcitonin) nasal spray, another commonly prescribed treatment, needs more proof that it prevents fractures. (As you analyze information about new drugs for osteoporosis, look at whether it prevents fracture, not just what it does to bone density tests. Some drugs may build bone back but it may not be the good quality of bone that was there originally and this cannot be measured by bone density tests).

Other biphosphonates are under development and may be hitting the market in the next few years. The important point to make is that osteoporosis has always been at least in part preventable, but now it's also *treatable.* This is a major change. As women move inexorably toward the age of fracture risk, these developments couldn't come too soon. But you would rather avoid the risk altogether by getting your bones as strong as possible now.

Two developments are very recent. A biphosphonate like Fosamax named zoledronic acid may be given once a year or less intravenously and stabilizes the bone mass. For example, it will be given in one dose when a woman is in the hospital for a hip fracture. The FDA approval is probably 5 years away. Very recently, pulsed or intermittent doses of parathyroid hormone—a hormone that usually results in resorption of normal bone—has been shown to restore bone mass and very effectively prevents fractures. This must be injected daily and can be taken for up to 24 months. The FDA approved this drug November 2002. It is named teriparatide, brand name Forteo.

What Should I Do Now?
No matter what age you are now, you should assess your own risks for osteoporosis. If you are Caucasian or Asian, if you drink or smoke, if you are slender in build, if you have a sedentary lifestyle and most importantly if you have a family history of osteoporosis and fractures, you are at high risk. You should go to your doctor and ask him or her to do a bone mineral density measurement. For more information, look at

the National Osteoporosis Foundation website, www.nof.org.

Next look at everything you may be doing right and anything you may be doing wrong and begin changing things. Osteoporosis is one of those quiet killers and worse yet, it usually makes you suffer a good deal before it finally finishes you off with that terminal hip fracture. Do you really want to be a crooked old lady with the so-called "Dowager's Hump" or what we call kyphosis?

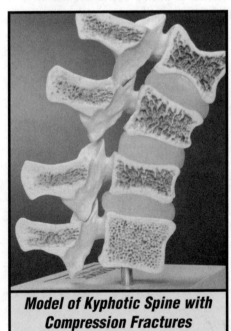

Model of Kyphotic Spine with Compression Fractures

A Few Words on Kyphosis

If you're having trouble seeing yourself as an old lady lying in bed with a broken hip, perhaps you can see yourself as bent over with kyphosis.

This deformity occurs through a gradual loss of bone mass in the vertebral skeleton, leading to multiple compression fractures of the vertebra. As these vertebrae collapse the spine gradually crumbles forward on itself, as the natural curves become accentuated. This is the source of the loss of height that naturally occurs with age, but it can be dramatic and painful in women with osteoporosis. Some get to the point where the rib cage is actually bent forward to the pelvis.

Kyphosis is not just the result of what my mother used to call "poor posture", but that is part of it. Many of us work in a head-forward, shoulder-hunched, slumped position for long hours. If this is not countered by stretching exercises of the anterior neck muscles and the pectoralis, or chest muscles, a person can, over time, develop this body configuration permanently. In that sense, my mother was right. "Sit up straight!" is still good advice.

At first the problem is only weak extensor muscles and tight flexor muscles with no underlying bony deformity. But as osteoporosis sneaks in, this "postural round back" may become a permanent bony kyphosis, as the upper thoracic vertebrae sustain silent compression fractures. The end result is the dowager's hump, and who wants that? I advise all of my patients in whom I detect this condition, or whose job predisposes them to develop it, to do the following exercises on a daily basis.

First, stretch your anterior neck muscles by turning your head fully from side to side several times. Then stretch your chest muscles by rolling your outstretched arms backwards in arm circles. In addition, it is important to strengthen your rhomboid muscles, the small thick muscles that hold the shoulder blades together. The best and simplest exercise for this is to bend at the waist while holding light hand weights, 2 to 5 pounds, and then raise your outstretched arms up until they are parallel with the floor. Then slowly release them downward again.

Another exercise that is helpful as a break after prolonged periods of sitting in a head-forward position is as follows. Stand at the corner of a wall and press both palms on either side of the corner at shoulder level. Then lean into the corner while arching the head and the spine. This rebalances the muscles of the upper back and neck and is a relaxing exercise.

When my wife's mother was forty-five, she enrolled in an aerobics class. In 1975, women did not know about osteoporosis or calcium deficiency and were just beginning to believe they should exercise. She had five children and had breast-fed all of them, giving away a substantial amount of her own calcium. After two weeks in aerobics, she complained of back pain. The complaint persisted so she had an x-ray of her lumbar spine. She had two lumbar compression fractures, the type of spine fractures that do not displace but are most commonly associated with osteoporosis. This was her wake-up call. She now takes 1500 mg. of calcium daily and estrogen replacement medication, and has had no further fractures.

Her experience probably strengthened the bones of her three daughters because they all became immediately aware of their own inadequate calcium intake and their genetic predisposition to osteoporosis.

The Future Comes to the Office with Her Mother

So often I see the devastation that Mom's final hip fracture visits on the family. Just last week, into my office rolled a tall, thin white-haired, blue-eyed 85 year-old woman. She was in a wheelchair and one month out from her hip fracture. In the hospital her surgery had gone fine but her recovery was complicated by a prolonged period of mental confusion that was just now clearing. But it was also clear that Mom was never going to be her complete self again. Around 50% of women who break their hips will never get back to same level of function they enjoyed before the break, regardless of how well-treated it is, how well it heals or how vigorous the

284

rehabilitation. Pushing Mom's wheelchair was her daughter, a slender, graying blonde-haired chip off the old block. I could see in the daughter's pale blue eyes the stresses of that last month and the vision of her own future that she was wheeling into my clinic. Everything she wanted for her mother's well-being was doubly heartfelt in that she was seeing herself twenty or thirty years from now. I thought, "You know, now I have two patients."

And that's the lesson for midlife women. Get with program right now. Look at what you can do to prevent osteoporosis if you haven't got it yet. If you have been through or are going through menopause, talk to your doctor about what you might do to halt the inevitable slide toward osteoporosis. And if you already think you may have it, but haven't had a fracture yet, get a bone mineral density test and avail yourself of the bone restorative treatments that are now available. Finally, talk with your daughters right now about what they can be doing to break the chain and avoid breaking their hips.

Chapter 14:
Miscellaneous
Orthopedic Conditions
(I Wouldn't Wish on My Worst Enemy)

Not all orthopedic conditions fit into some anatomic, regional classification. Some of the worst problems we see are what we call "systemic" diseases. This means they affect either the whole body or some whole organ system, in this case, all the joints at once or all the bones at once. The classic example of a systemic disease that affects all the joints at once is rheumatoid arthritis, which I've already discussed (*Chapter 3: Arthritis*). Now let's look at gout and then bone and joint infections, and tumors of the bones and joints.

Uncle Woody's Got the Gout

"Gout, unlike any other disease, kills more rich men than poor, more wise men than simple. Great kings, emperors, generals, admirals and philosophers have all died of gout."

Thomas Sydenham 1624-1689

Gout, often called the "disease of kings," is related to overdoing of all kinds: being over-weight, over-eating and heavy drinking. In that sense it might be a prototypic boomer disease—-too much of a good thing. Gout results when the body suffers from too much of the waste product called uric acid. Uric acid comes from the metabolism of certain foods called "purines," generally rich foods that come from animal organs like brains, livers, sweetbreads, kidneys and other decadent stuff. You know, the kind of stuff British people like to eat. Purines also come naturally from the breakdown of the body's own cells. Uric acid levels can rise above normal from the over-consumption of certain rich foods, from the changes brought about by heavy drinking, and at times from problems certain people have with clearing uric acid through their kidneys. When the concentration of uric acid in the blood reaches a certain critical level, it begins to precipitate out in the joint fluid as a crystal, causing an intense inflammatory response, pain and swelling. The joints just do not like uric acid crystals irritating the synovium.

How to Avoid or Limit Gout

- Avoid purine-rich foods like beer, wine and other alcoholic drinks, anchovies, sardines in oil, fish roes, herring, yeast, organ meats (liver, kidneys, etc.), legumes like dried beans, peas, meat extracts, consommé, gravies, mushrooms, spinach, asparagus, cauliflower and poultry.
- Be careful of certain diuretic medications like thiazide.
- Seek treatment for kidney disorders that impair the body's clearance of these purines.
- Once diagnosed with gout, you may need suppressive medication (allopurinol).

Commonly, gout attacks at night, and it is much more common in men than in women. So, a modern version of Shakespeare's gouty Falstaff character would be Uncle Woody who's staying over Thanksgiving night, sleeping off the abundance of the harvest feast. Let's say he had about a bottle and a half of red wine over the course of the day. Oh, he loved the creamed herring and, yes, he had seconds on the liver and scallops and the sweatbreads. (These may not be your usual Thanksgiving meal but they are foods rich in purines, sure to cause an attack of gout.) Uncle Woody fell asleep around 8:00 PM in the evening after we'd all decided it just wasn't safe for the oversized man to drive home. He was still snoring when the rest of the family turned in around 11:00 PM.

But around 4:00 AM Woody awakens with a stabbing pain in his big toe. He stumbles into your john in search of at least Tylenol, but he would settle for some Percodan if you have any. When you look at his toe, it is red, swollen, and excruciatingly tender. Woody has "the gout."

It's Not So Great Being the King

Though we usually think of gout as affecting the bunion joint or other small joints in the foot, it can affect any joint. It commonly chooses the large joints like the knee and ankle, and occasionally the wrist and hand. In severe cases, it can affect several joints at once. The treatment is first to recognize it. This is easy when it shows up in the bunion of a big fat slob with alcohol on his breath, but the diagnosis can be more subtle when it presents in a woman's wrist. In cases of gout, when a uric acid level is drawn from the blood, it is usually elevated—but not always. Occasionally, the doctor will have to needle and aspirate the joint itself and send the joint fluid to the lab to be tested for uric acid crystals. Once the diagnosis is confirmed, the patient is treated with strong anti-inflammatory drugs like cortisone, indomethacin and sometimes a drug called colchicine, which has been around for years. In patients who have repeated attacks that aren't controlled by dietary moderation, a drug called Allopurinol (zyloprim) is added. This suppresses the attacks by keeping the body from building up uric acid.

In the worst cases, gouty collections can accumulate under the skin in little lumpy nodules called "tophi," not to be confused with "tofu," which is something that gout-ridden people would never even consider eating. I see gout all the time in the clinic and it is a diagnosis commonly missed by primary care doctors. It can look so much like an infected joint, which is a serious condition, that patients with that diagnosis are usually referred for emergency treatment. Though not a surgical emergency, like an infected joint, the gouty joint is no less distressing to the patient and no less in need of immediate, aggressive treatment. So, even though the patient has been sent to me for the wrong reason, he gets correctly diagnosed and receives the help he needs. Right church; wrong pew. How people suffered through the ages with this condition is truly the subject of folklore. Risk factors for gout read like a list of well-he-just-let-himself-go conditions: hypertension, alcoholism, obesity, diabetes, hyperlipidemia (too much fat in your blood), immobility etc. No wonder this has historically been considered a disease of the upper classes.

No one who is taking reasonable care of himself is likely to suffer from gout, unless he has some genetically determined metabolic screw-up that interferes with his handling the normal excretion of uric acid. So, even though this may be the only condition for which you can count yourself in the company of Benjamin Franklin and Thomas Jefferson, it's still nothing to be proud of.

When Osteoarthritis Masquerades as King: Pseudogout

Gout is the classic example of what we call a "crystalline" arthritis, literally an arthritis where the joint inflammation is caused by some crystal precipitating in the joint. In the case of gout, the crystal is uric acid salt. However, there is another common form of crystalline arthritis that occurs in patients with garden-variety osteoarthritis. This is called "pseudogout," and, as the name implies, it looks a lot like gout. Pseudogout is caused by a precipitation of the local calcium and phosphate minerals released in the breakdown of the joint that occurs during joint degeneration. These gather together into a very irritating crystal that arouses an inflammation that mimics gout, but is usually not quite so bad. Because of the calcium involved, pseudogout causes a characteristic appearance on the x-ray that makes the diagnosis easier, as long as the doctor is at least looking for it. Pseudogout is also treated with anti-inflammatory drugs, and responds very nicely to cortisone injections into the affected joint.

Musculoskeletal Infections

Man lives in harmony with more microorganisms and little animals than you could possibly imagine. There are bugs on our skin and in every orifice. There are tiny mites in our eyelashes and hordes of bacteria in our intestines. Every human, no matter how tidy he may believe himself to be, is, in fact, a cottage industry of bacteria, viruses and other little creatures who are mostly along for the ride and are, by and large, pretty well-behaved. Like it or not, we have evolved together and there's just no evicting them from the apartment. But every now and then, the human defenses break down and the bugs win out; they get into where they're not supposed to be or they replicate in greater numbers than is good for the boomer host. We call this state an "infection." The two significant musculoskeletal infections are osteomyelitis (infection in the bone) and septic arthritis (infection in the joint). I will discuss the bacterial version of each, but there are more obscure bone and joint infections caused by viruses and even worms and other parasites.

Osteomyelitis

An infection in the substance of the bone is called "osteomyelitis" and it is a very serious condition. Osteomyelitis can be caused by blood-borne bacteria settling into the bone from some distant source (such as an abscessed tooth or a kidney infection), or from direct inoculation into an open fracture. Bone is actually very resistant to infection, because of its limited blood supply, but this advantage becomes a disadvantage once an active bone infection is established. It is very difficult to eradicate bone infections because bone turnover is slow, and because the blood supply is so limited. Orthopedists have a saying: "Osteomyelitis is forever." It is not unusual to see a bone infection lay dormant for years only to reactivate with some stress such as surgery on the adjacent tissues.

Boomers are usually spared the blood-borne (we call this "hematogenous") form of osteomyelitis, because it more commonly occurs in infants and old folks. This is the same as saying it occurs when the immune system is either immature or played out. For this same reason, people with immune deficiencies like AIDS, or those induced in the treatment of cancer or the suppression of rejection in transplant patients, are prone to osteomyelitis. The same holds true for joint infections. Boomers tend to get osteomyelitis that starts with some catastrophic open fracture. Tibia fractures are especially prone to this, occurring as they do during high velocity trauma and in an area without much soft tissue covering the bone.

Once established, osteomyelitis causes deep pain in the bone, often worse at night. There will be localized tenderness over the affected area, usually redness and fever. If left untreated, eventually the bone abscess may seek to drain itself and erupt to the surface as a draining sinus tract. When chronic, there are typical signs on the bone x-ray and blood tests that show marked elevations in the parameters that signal a serious infection.

The treatment is open biopsy and culture of the affected part of the bone, drainage of the pus and removal of any dead bone, followed by a very long course of antibiotics, usually given through the veins. The culture of the specific bacteria causing the infection is critical to choosing the proper antibiotic. Repeated surgeries are often necessary to make sure the infected bone tissue is cleaned up and allowed to heal.

By now you get the idea that osteomyelitis is a horrible affliction and, once established, the patient is in for the battle of his life. Though modern antibiotics have made the treatment of many of these infections more effective, the bugs are fighting back with increasing resistance. The overuse and casual misuse of "big gun" antibiotics for every little sniffle and dribble has backfired, driving some previously innocent bacteria into a life of crime.

Septic Arthritis

Infection in a joint is just as serious as infection in the bone, but for a different reason. Joint infections may destroy the articular cartilage and lead rapidly to severe arthritis. The same bacteria that infect bones can infect joints, both from hematogenous sources and direct inoculation. Like osteomyelitis, septic arthritis is also more common at both ends of the age spectrum and when the immune system is depressed or impaired. Joint infections are easier to cure, though, because the joint lining has a rich blood supply and, therefore, antibiotics can easily be delivered to the location of the infection.

Where osteomyelitis and septic arthritis differ most is in the urgency of treatment. If unrecognized or untreated, an infection will destroy the joint cartilage in a matter of hours, certainly within a few days. Osteomyelitis can smolder for quite some time and the outcome of treatment will likely be no different than if promptly recognized, but neglect a septic joint over the weekend and that joint is dead forever. We consider septic arthritis in a major joint to be a surgical emergency. We wash the pus out of the joint immediately, either by opening the joint or, sometimes, through smaller incisions with the arthroscope.

You may notice that I haven't tried to add much humor to this section and that's because there is just nothing at all funny about either osteomyelitis or septic arthritis. Worldwide, these two conditions taken together are probably *the* most common orthopedic problem, especially in the so-called "developing" countries. The scariest part is the emergence of antibiotic-resistant organisms, especially new varieties of tuberculosis and a few others for which we really have no effective antibiotic defenses. We forget that in the generation before ours, the great global plague was the viral, neuromuscular infection poliomyelitis. A whole generation of orthopedists was trained to treat the victims of polio. My great fear is that somewhere out there a robust, resistant bacterium is evolving; one that eats our antibiotics like candy and prefers the bones and joints. I want to be retired when that sucker comes along.

Bone Tumors

I'm not going to try to cover the whole waterfront of musculoskeletal tumors, but rather to make a few general comments. First, there are benign tumors of the bone and then there are the malignant tumors. The benign tumors, which are common, may cause fractures by weakening the bone. For this reason, they may present as calamities. But they are usually short-term calamities. The malignant tumors can be thought of as two varieties. First, there are those that arise primarily in the bone from one of the normal cells that make up bone. Here it gets a little complicated. "Bone cell" refers to the osteocytes alone, the cell that makes bone and is the primary cell in bone. But there are also blood-making cells (marrow cells) in bone, blood vessel cells (in the blood vessels within bone), nerve cells (in the nerves within bone), fibrous tissue cells and even little muscle cells in the vessel walls within bone. Any of these cells can go awry and cause a cancer. Worse yet, since any cell anywhere contains the genetic permission to be any other cell in the human body, a cell can "de-differentiate" and transform itself from a bone cell to, say, a cartilage cell and make a cartilage tumor within the bone. So I used the term "cells in bone" with a purpose. If I say just "bone cells" it implies that all malignancies arise from the osteocyte[15] cell line alone, which is far from the case. Perhaps, "cells that make up bone" is more accurate. These are called "primary" bone tumors and are actually pretty rare. The second group of malignant bone arise elsewhere and then settle into the bone. These are called "metastatic" tumors and have behaviors characteristic of the cancer from which they came.

The most common primary bone tumors are actually not bone cell tumors at all, but blood cell malignancies that arise from the marrow inhabitants of bone. We call these

15 The osteocyte is the main bone cell; the cell that manufactures and maintains all the structural elements of bone.

"hematopoetic" tumors, meaning that they arise in the cells that are part of the blood system, not of the bone itself. These may be from the lymph cells (lymphomas), from the plasma cells (multiple myeloma), or from the white blood cells (leukemias). None of these are good news, but none is the death sentence that it used to be. The trick for the orthopedist is to maintain an awareness that these conditions are out there and may mimic infections or other conditions. We have another saying: "Biopsy all infections; culture all tumors." What this means is that I can be looking at an x-ray or lab work, and be ready to treat a lesion that for all the world looks like it ought to be an infection—and it's actually a malignancy. Conversely, I may be fooled by what looks exactly like a malignancy, when, in fact, it's an osteomyelitis.

Certain cancers have a propensity to spread to bone. These include malignancies of the lung, breast, kidney, thyroid and prostate. These five account for the overwhelming majority of metastatic tumors that we see. They usually cause either fractures or impending fractures by replacing the normal bone elements with cancer cells. The average orthopedist may see one or two primary bone tumors in his career, but he will see many metastatic lesions and probably quite a few hematopoetic malignancies affecting the bone.

Of all the above, I am most likely to see a boomer woman with metastatic breast cancer, either a man or woman with metastatic lung cancer and more rarely someone with multiple myeloma, a blood cell tumor that affects many bones at the same time. I'm most likely to be called upon to stabilize a weakened bone; either one that is riddled with cancer cells and about to fracture, or one that already has broken through. We are usually able to either stabilize the broken bone, or, when the fracture is near a major joint like the hip or shoulder, replace the whole joint with a prosthesis, discarding the cancer in the bargain. Though there is a whole sub-specialty of orthopedists trained in the treatment of what we call "musculoskeletal oncology," they are few and far between. They are a rare breed mostly inhabiting the ivory towers, medical schools and large private clinics like Mayo Clinic, M. D. Anderson in Houston, the Cleveland Clinic and the Ochsner Clinic where I work. Frontline orthopedists send those rare primary bone tumors to them for the latest treatment, but there's way too much metastatic bone disease for that to be treated only by these sub-specialists. The average orthopedist is usually quite competent and experienced in the treatment of those metastatic tumors that weaken the bone.

I titled this chapter "Miscellaneous Orthopedic Conditions (That I Wouldn't Wish on My Worst Enemy)" knowing that would be about the last clever thing I would be able to squeeze in. The collective misery of gout, osteomyelitis, septic arthritis and bone tumors is just not a subject for a lot of yucks. Throughout the ages it has been the trauma of the battlefield, the everyday fractures and these miserable conditions that have made orthopedics a specialty unto itself. It is only very recently that we've had the luxury of focusing on such fine arts as joint replacement, hand surgery or something ultimately as vain and frivolous as "sports medicine." Even into the last half of the 20th century, we were mostly setting fractures, draining pus, passing out canes and going to funerals. I hope we never lose sight of how much we've elevated our game. We have unintentionally fostered an attitude that suggests we can cure anything, straighten anything that's crooked, fix anything that's broken, cut out what shouldn't be there and erase the ravages of time. The truth is we are still almost completely powerless in the face of a truly aggressive malignancy. We don't even understand what causes rheumatoid arthritis, and we still have a hell of a time getting rid of bone infections. I wouldn't wish any of these conditions on my worst enemy.

Chapter 15: The Paradoxes

Paradox comes from the Greek word for "incredible." In this book I pose some questions whose answers seem paradoxical. For example, even though I am a surgeon, in many cases I advise against surgery. In some cases I advise exercise as a treatment and in other cases I incriminate it as a prime cause of injury. What gives? How can these paradoxes be resolved? Is there some middle ground— some compromise? My response is, "That's it! You've seen the light!" The answer to the treatment of many medical problems is almost always the middle ground. For action-oriented boomers this sort of resolution is counter-intuitive, unnatural and out of character. By nature we are not compromisers, or middle-seekers.

I want to take you through these paradoxes as I understand them and to prescribe what I see as the resolution for each one. I have grouped them artificially into four categories: the exercise paradoxes; the surgical paradoxes; the sports paradoxes; and the paradoxes of evolution. I say "artificially" because they are all obviously interrelated and can't be completely teased out into these neat little categories. But in a world of "lumpers" and "splitters," I'm a born lumper.

The Exercise Paradoxes

"Exercise is good, but too much exercise is bad." All the syndromes except deconditioning fall prey to this paradox. The best example is the stress fracture caused by excessive, repetitive loading of a long bone. You remember the "Fear-of-becoming-a-Fat Lady" Syndrome, the woman who pounds her hips to death on the treadmill, or the "Fitness-is-Competition" Syndrome guy who trains for the Iron Man

harder and longer until eventually his tibia breaks. These stress fractures are *always* preceded by pain in the bone that gradually gets worse with exercise. Ignoring pain on the mistaken notion that "no pain; no gain" is nonsense. Increasing or persistent pain is always a warning sign. Persistent pain deserves prompt evaluation. Period. It may be nothing, but how do you know that without asking someone who can actually answer the question, such as your doctor? And he or she may not be able to give you a definitive answer without an x-ray and sometimes without a bone scan or an MRI.

Any exercise can be overdone. If someone comes to me and complains that he's having shoulder pain only after the second mile he swims, I'm naturally going to ask him, "Why the hell are you swimming two miles?" If he says, "I'm getting ready for a triathlon," I'm going to say, "Get a life! How about settling for the 6K?" I'm glad there are boomers who can do triathlons, but most of us can't and shouldn't— *and* we shouldn't feel badly about it.

A good rule of thumb to follow is: any exercise that hurts you probably isn't good for you. Call that "Wilson's Rule," if you like, but for any exercise that's causing you pain, I'll bet I can think of a substitute that won't. And so can you, if you keep your mind open. A corollary of this is that any exercise that doesn't hurt can be taken to an extreme that will eventually harm you. I'm reminded of my friend who wasn't satisfied cycling centuries (100 miles at a time); he had to work up to riding 200 and then 300 miles in one day! Guess what? He just about killed himself and had to stop riding for quite some time.

Exercise should be fun, but even when it isn't, it should at least be sensible.

"Jogging may be good for your heart, yet bad for your joints." This one is sad but true. In general, running is the most convenient aerobic activity available. It requires almost no equipment other than the right shoes and some open road. It is quick, portable, variable and good for your heart, and yet it's absolute punishment for your knees, back, neck and feet. I'm happy for that small percentage of people who are able to jog, but as you get deeper into the midlife years, the damage starts to add up. Eventually roadrunners will have some kind of orthopedic problem that brings them down. It may be temporary, it may be minor, or it may be the final straw. I think every jogger should be thinking about plan B. In fact, the smartest thing of all is to do some sort of cross-training that mixes a few jogs a week with other non-impact aerobic activities such as brisk walking, treadmill, cycling, swimming etc.

I remember cycling in the Hill Country north of San Antonio, Texas with two of my residents in the early 1990s. I was in my early forties then. We closed head-on with a middle-aged jogger who was bow-legged, flat-footed and flailing along with one arm jerking one way and one arm swinging the other. He ran like Joe Cocker sings. He was grinding up the same hill we were sailing down, and he was obviously in great pain. As we breezed by this Apparition of Fitness Past, one of my residents said, "You just don't get any style points for joggin'."

If you've jogged all your life, don't stop now, but make some plans for what you're going to do when you no longer can. Better yet, start to ease into those alternatives sooner, before you do irreparable damage.

Treadmills may be boring but they are much better for your joints. Put some weights in your hands if you want a more aerobic challenge. Put the treadmill in front of the VCR and get some interesting tapes to watch. The newer "elliptical" exercisers are also very easy on most joints and are a very low impact way of keeping in shape. These are the machines where your feet progress around in, essentially, an elliptical arc; they are a blend of the steppers, ski machines and treadmills.

Just remember, every time you escape Earth's gravitational pull and come back to ground, you're asking your knees, your back, your feet and your future to absorb the shock.

"Chronic problems have chronic solutions." This principle doesn't even sound like a paradox, but you'd be surprised at how much time I spend trying to explain this simple axiom of rehabilitation to my patients. Boomers want quick, definitive remedies, not life-style changes or philosophical advice. Whenever I prescribe exercises as therapy for some condition, I try to explain to people that there are three reasons why people fail physical therapy. They all are my fault, if I don't warn you. So here goes.

The first reason for failure is that when you start an exercise program, the muscle or joint you're exercising usually hurts a little more in the beginning, so many people stop right there. Now I'm *not* talking about "hurts a lot for a long time," just that little "spring training effect" that goes along with any new exercise program—the kind of ache that will go away in a week or less if you keep up a low level, gentle program. This is the excuse the whimps use when they say they tried therapy and it didn't work. "It made me worse!" The answer here is to just keep up with the program at a beginner's level for a little longer. Eventually, those start-up pains will usually just resolve. If they don't, then this is probably a warning sign. Either the doctor has prescribed the wrong exercise, has the wrong diagnosis or the therapist is overdoing it.

The second reason for failure is keeping up with an exercise program for a while, but not long enough for it to have the intended impact. If someone comes to me with six months of shoulder pain from rotator cuff weakness, I don't really expect to see a response to the exercises within the first few weeks. I explain that it may well be months before they see any sign of improvement, so just hang in there.

The third and final reason for failure is when a person does the exercises long enough that they have the desired effect, but then stops doing them, thinking that the problem is behind them—gone for good. Chronic problems have chronic solutions. This is especially true for most shoulder problems, back pain and some types of knee pain. The solution is all about maintenance. It's like brushing your teeth; you just have to keep doing it.

So whether you're assessing your current exercise program, trying to design a new one, or have just had one prescribed as therapy for some orthopedic ailment, start with low or no impact activities that you enjoy. Then mix it up; don't get stuck with just one exercise regimen. Think of what you're doing as maintenance of the machine, not competition or physical sculpture. Perform your workout either where you are or where you like to be. For some people (like me) that means at home; for others, that means the gym. For some it's outdoors; for others it's behind closed doors.

Remember: pain is almost always a warning sign and very few people can run marathons.

The Surgical Paradoxes

"Some surgeries make you worse more often than they make you better." It may seem paradoxical to have a guy who makes his living as a surgeon telling you that there are operations that have a questionable justification, or what we call in our jargon "limited indications." I've alluded to most of these as we've discussed the various joints, fractures and the spine. The best example of a questionable indication for surgery is almost any surgery directed exclusively at back pain. Remember: surgery on the spine directed at relieving leg pain from pinched nerves is predictable, effective and worth considering. Surgery offered simply for back pain—no matter what the supposed justification (degenerated discs, spinal instability etc)—is just as likely to be either ineffective or even to make the situation worse.

The same can be said for some of the newer, "less-invasive" procedures such as endoscopic carpal tunnel release or any of a number of arthroscopic procedures. In my book, for any less invasive procedure to meet muster it must fulfill all of the following criteria:

- *It must be able to accomplish what it's supposed to do at least as well as the open procedure it proposes to displace. A smaller scar is little solace if you don't get the job done.*

- *The recovery from the less invasive procedure must be shorter, less painful or in some way enhanced, compared to the standard procedure.*

- *The surgery itself should take no more than twice as long as the open procedure. Sound funny? In the early days of arthroscopic shoulder surgery, for*

*instance, the surgeon would often rummage
around with the arthroscope for an hour or
two, and then abandon the attempt, open the
shoulder and do whatever he was up to "the
old fashioned" way.*

Here we're back to the old adage of asking your surgeon why he's recommending this type of surgery over another type, how many he's done this way and, basically, "What's in it for me?" There are absolute masters of arthroscopic surgery out there—guys who can do an arthroscopic rotator cuff repair in an hour and lop off the end of an arthritic clavicle to boot. You should feel perfectly comfortable accepting their recommendations. But if someone tells you that he's done ten, they've all taken at least three hours, and 50% of the time he has to open them anyway, sign up for his open repair and skip the learning curve. What's important is that the rotator cuff gets sewn back to the humerus, not the length of the incision.

"'Cutting edge' and 'state-of-the-art' is not always what you want." We are a culture of technology junkies, and orthopedists are some of the biggest junkies of all. We are like packrats: we're attracted to bright shiny objects. I saw a wonderful demonstration of this a few years ago when I was helping my wife Kathy teach the management of musculoskeletal problems to a group of internists. Internists don't think or act like orthopedists; they just don't. I was giving my lectures over the lunch hour and had been hitting up the local pharmaceutical companies to put on the feed-bag. I'm telling trade secrets here, but docs call these "drug lunches." Well, I ran the deck on the *Searles* and the *Pfizers*, and, finally, I asked one of our orthopedic equipment companies—the guys who make the implants we use—to do the lunch. They gladly did, and if I did 400 of your implants

a year, you would too. Since I was going to speak on the knee, I asked the equipment guy to bring in the instruments we use for doing a total knee replacement. This stuff looks like toolbox after toolbox of cutting jigs, alignment jigs, and trial implants—your basic surgical Home Depot, aisle number four.

The internists looked at this paraphernalia as if it was radioactive. As they piled their plates with bowtie pasta, they skirted the surgical hardware as if it would explode in their hands, if they so much as picked it up. I had two of my residents with me that day, and, of course, they walked right up to the trays full of metal parts, parked their bagels between their teeth and started playing with everything they could get both mitts on. Even though they'd seen all this stuff a hundred times before, they still had to touch it, lift it, move anything with moving parts, un-screw anything that came apart and then screw it back together again.

That, in a nutshell, is our mentality. We are gadgeteers of the highest order. And because of this, we are suckers for the latest, greatest technological change. Notice I didn't say "advance." We often don't know whether any given change is an advance until it has proven itself over ten years. This is especially true in joint replacement, a field where everything looks good at first but where long-term durability is the name of the game. I teach my residents, "Beware the 'state-of-the-art!' We often don't know what knuckleheads we are for five or ten years." I'm embarrassed to say that I can give you numerous examples of changes that were touted as "state-of-the-art," the "latest advance," or the "current trend," and then over time proved to be unmitigated disasters. We are forever climbing out on what we think is the main limb of the tree of orthopedic evolution, only to saw it off behind ourselves and come crashing back to earth.

For example, we've changed the polyethylene—the plastic bearing in joint replacements—and sometimes we've made it better. But just as often we've made it worse. We've tried artificial ligaments, and joint replacements for joints that were too small for them to hold up. We tried to do away with bone cement and then brought it back, singing its praises. My point is that doctors have to be careful not to accept all changes as advances, and so you should be careful too. Be cautious about what you hear on the tube, read in the paper or hear at the gym. You want to know about the science behind each new procedure and the track record behind the next so-called miracle.

I've had that kind of nutty patient who's crazy about new surgical procedures. Let's say about ten years ago he had two hip replacements done by one of my predecessors, and I do the follow-up examinations on him. He's doing fine, but every year when he comes in for his checkup, he always asks about the latest advances and "what's new on the horizon." This year he's having trouble with his back and wants me to refer him to "somebody on the cutting edge." He looks at my handsome twenty-eight-year-old intern with exactly six weeks total experience in orthopedics and says, "You know, somebody like him. Not somebody gray like you." He is dead serious. The cruel joke is that patients with this attitude often get both what they want and exactly what they deserve.

As a patient, what you need to ask is "How long has this procedure been around? What are the usual short-term *and* long-term results? Has this procedure even been around long enough for us to *know* the long-term results?" For the record, we call the first two years after a joint replacement "short-term follow-up." From three to five years is considered an "intermediate term follow-up." And we don't consider a procedure a "long term follow-up" until the ten-year mark. That's why we don't know what knuckleheads we are for at least ten years. Would you want a joint replacement that looked good at two years, not so good at five, and then failed miserably before ten years was out?

"I'm a surgeon who frequently advises against surgery." The busier you are as a surgeon, the more conservative you become. Many conditions have a surgical solution, but even in my business, these are far from the majority. Most conditions can and should be treated without surgery. I think of surgery as the last choice for any problem, and you should too. Surgery is a decision arrived at only after thinking through all other possibilities and exhausting all other alternatives. If both surgeons and patients can cultivate this attitude, we will be keeping to the first principle of all medical practice (attributed to Hippocrates): "In the first place, do no harm."

This isn't to say that there aren't conditions where doctors think first of surgery—open fractures, for instance—because we know that there are no reasonable alternatives. Many mechanical problems have mechanical solutions. A torn meniscus usually will not heal on its own and, therefore, arthroscopic trimming of the torn part is the best answer. Complete rotator cuff tears also don't heal by themselves, and all surgeons would agree that these need to be repaired surgically. But in each case the decision for surgery is based on the physician's understanding of the injury or the disease process, its behavior and potential for healing, and the probable success of surgery. For most patients in the boomer age group, the risk factors associated with the patient's general health are not a big issue, but with the elderly patient, poor health may render a surgical solution completely out of the question.

Here again, the patient and the surgeon may have conflicting expectations and goals that come into direct conflict. The boomer patient almost always wants the quickest, most direct solution to whatever problem is bringing him to me. He or she is usually in the "prime of life," which today means working one or more jobs, putting two or more kids through college and just overall trying to stay afloat in this sea of chaos. The boomer with an orthopedic problem may come to my office with an unrealistic faith in technology and surgery, and a well-read but at least partially misinformed notion of his problem. So he may already have decided that he needs this or that surgery to get back in the game. His attitude is somewhere in the neighborhood of, "If we can put a man on the moon, why can't you just operate on my elbow and take away this pain?"

But the smart surgeon knows that even the simplest operation can go awry. Any incision can become infected, anything sewn together can fall apart, and anything straightened out can go crooked. Not all fractures heal. Every artificial implant in the human body will eventually fail, unless you fail before it does. And so it goes. My job is to make sure you understand what you're asking for (in the case of elective surgery) or getting into (in the case of emergency surgery). We call this "informed consent," but it boils down to making sure the patient is informed enough to feel consensual.

Informed consent involves telling the patient about the chances—the statistical chances—of a reasonable outcome. Here we get into some great quotations, including Mark Twain's famous line about, "lies, damn lies and statistics." I really like what Thomas Carlyle (1795-1881) said:

> "A judicious man looks at statistics, not to get knowledge, but to save himself from having

309

ignorance foisted on him."

If you ask me, "What are my chances of getting an infection with this total knee replacement, Doc?" I will answer, "Less than one percent." But, in fact, what I'm thinking to myself is more like, "Well, for *you*, my friend, the chance is actually 50-50, since the statistical chance of any one occurrence is the same as the flip of a coin—it will either happen or it won't. But if you're smart, you'll choose to look at yourself as one patient in a hundred having this operation and in that case, your chances are less than one in a hundred."

I use this same principle in reverse when I want to scare someone off from an operation I don't think they should have. When they ask, "What is the chance this operation will be a success, Doc?" I say, "Probably no better than 50-50." And I say it with a straight face, because I'm telling the God's honest truth. For my money, the best quotation for this situation is from that most prolific of all authors, Anonymous:

> *"Medical statistics are like a bikini. What they reveal is interesting but what they conceal is vital."*

Remember that you're coming to the doctor for his opinion. Don't be so inflexible that you shut off the discussion as soon as you hear something that contradicts your expectation. We are, after all, having a discussion, up to the point where we decide together how to proceed. Sometimes we'll proceed with pills; sometimes with physical therapy; sometimes with surgery. But the "we" is the key. I'm going to tell you what I think, give you some choices and as much information as time permits—though in modern medicine that never seems to be enough, but that's another story. If surgery is the only way to go, it should be an easy decision. If the decision seems difficult, then surgery is probably not the best answer.

The Sports Paradox

"The sports that were fun at 20 may be dangerous at 50."
This paradox is at the very heart of the Fitness-Is-Competition Syndrome and the Risk-Taker Syndrome, but it can just as easily sneak up and whack the weekend skier or the guy who decides to play in the company softball league. Look in the mirror. Lots of things have changed in the thirty years between Viet Nam and September 11th, not the least of which are your flexibility, your reflexes and your ability to recover from injury. When I was in the Air Force, we used to have a yearly softball game between the orthopedic doctors and the clinic staff. We were mostly in our thirties and forties; they were mostly in their twenties. I'm sure in our prime we could have whipped their butts, but in reality we usually injured ourselves. One year we had a hand surgeon who broke his ankle over-running a blooper into centerfield, a sports medicine guy who popped a hamstring trying to stretch a double, and two guys who hurt their fingers. This might sound comical, but as one of the "lucky" ones who didn't get dinged, I had to pull call twice as often, with my fellow Keystone Cops out on "injured reserve." This is not to mention the lost productivity of several surgeons being unable to meet muster. In fact, prior to the First Gulf War, the number one threat to the mission in the USAF was—you guessed it—softball!

I've already touched on this in several chapters. I've told you about the guy who tore his ACL in a pick-up basketball game, and the cyclist who broke his collarbone or worse yet, suffered a closed head injury. I've warned you that when you can *feel the wind in your hair,* you may be at risk for that Life-altering Event.

I honestly think that boomers have an obligation to their families, their employers, their employees and to society at large to stay healthy and to make sensible choices. Should you have a good time? Why, sure. I guess it was Thomas Jefferson who said that we were all entitled to "...life, liberty and the pursuit of happiness." But damn, he'd never seen a hang glider. As William Carlos Williams—a doctor as well as a poet—put it:

> *"so much depends*
> *upon*
> *a red wheel*
> *barrow*
> *glazed with rain*
> *water*
> *beside the white*
> *chickens"*

Don't look now, Bubba, but you are that red wheelbarrow! If you sprained your ankle while you were in college, it was an inconvenience getting to class. But if you tear up your rotator cuff playing racquetball now, you might not be able to take the time off you need to get over it. Can you afford—literally *afford*—to be out of commission for a few days at the time of surgery, in a sling for a month and in rehab for three to six months? I doubt it.

I'm not suggesting you take up chess, far from it. I'm counseling moderation. If you are going to choose competitive sports as one of your fitness pursuits, fine. Just don't go to the mat with it. Keep your eye on the ball: the goal is exercise and maintaining fitness. The goal is not "We're Number One!" If you're a competitor, it is far safer to compete with the computer in the StairMaster than with some young guy who reminds of you of your "Glory Days."

The Paradox of Evolution

I could put this paradox a couple of ways:

> *"If we're the crown of creation, why do we all have back pain?"*

> or

> *"I want to live to a hundred; how come I'm designed to live to thirty?"*

This is the one you probably don't want to think about, but this paradox underlies everything I've said. We are only on this planet for a brief time. Medical science and a higher standard of living may recently have extended that time a bit, but each of us is still an hourglass. Like it or not, the Wicked Witch of the East turned my hourglass over 50 years ago and, try as I might, I will never be able to turn it back. I could click the heels of my ruby slippers together over and over, but I will never escape my next birthday. I said in the *Introduction* that I made my living on the fringes of entropy, and I meant it. You can't fool Mother Nature, and your best bet is to take care of this body as well as you can for as long as you can. Try not to turn it from a temple into a trash can.

I think it's important to admit that we are just another one of God's creatures and, thereby, subject to all His natural laws. Our bones heal, but no better than your dog's. Our brain is a little bigger, but glance around the planet and it might be hard to say that's had such a positive effect. When someone asks me my "success rate" with, say, hip replacement, I answer, "Zero. Every one I've ever done will eventually fail." About all we can aspire to is good maintenance.

But I see good maintenance as an end in itself, and I hope I've given you some useful maintenance tips in this book. The boomer musculoskeletal system is fascinating, fun to deal with and still, in my mind at least, a real piece of work. I could quibble with God on some of the finer points of His design, but I'm going to lose that argument for sure. I still feel privileged that I have been able to help so many people keep their bones and joints functioning over the twenty-eight years I've been doing this. Still, I could use your help a little here. Some of you could make some smarter choices. If you're deconditioned, you could decide today to get off your butt and go for a walk. If you're constantly re-injuring yourself because you treasure competition above good sense, give it a rest. If you're worried that if you drop those twice-daily step-aerobics classes, you'll look less like Ali McBeal and more like Rosie O'Donell, fine. Just get your bone mineral density checked and have a hamburger now and then. If you want to look like Arnold Swartzennegger, ask him if he can order his shirts through *Land's End*. I'll bet he can't. Finally, if you like to *feel the wind in your hair,* please wear a helmet. Don't do it for me; do it for yourself.

Books by Whiskey Hollow Press:

The Other Midlife Crisis:
Arthritis and All Those Aches and Pains
By Michael R. Wilson, M.D., Orthopedic Surgeon

Dispatches From the Frontlines of Medicine:
Your Husband's Health:
Simplify Your Worry List
By Kathleen Wilson, M.D.

Coming Soon...

Dispatches From the Frontlines of Medicine:
By Kathleen Wilson, M.D.

For Women:
When You Feel Like You Are Falling Apart

Maintain Your Brain
Preventing Stroke and Dementia

When One Thing Leads to Another:
Critical Turning Points in the Health of Older Parents

Where is Marcus Welby When We Need Him?
Managing in the Medical System

Soul Survival:
Midlife Medicine for African Americans
By Giselle Wilson and Kathleen Wilson, M.D.

Midlife Medicine Series

Qty	Title	Price
	The Other Midlife Crisis: Arthritis and All Those Aches and Pains ISBN 0-9742976-0-7	$21.95
	Dispatches from the Frontlines of Medicine: Your Husband's Health: Simplify Your Worry List ISBN 0-9742976-1-5	$14.95
	Subtotal	
	Sales Tax (if applicable)	
	Shipping and Handling ($4.00 U.S./$14.00 International)	
	TOTAL	

Shipping Address

Name _____

Address _____

City_____ State_____ Zip Code_____

Country_____

Telephone_____ Fax_____ E-mail_____

Billing Address (if different from shipping)

Name _____

Address _____

City_____ State_____ Zip Code_____

Country_____

Name as it appears on your credit card_____

Credit card#_____cid#_____

Order by fax, mail or online:

Whiskey Hollow Press
P.O. Box 13752 • New Orleans, LA 70185-3752
(504) 861-2188 • Fax (504) 861-1657
www.boomermedicine.com
www.whiskeyhollowpress.com

Shipping time is usually 3-5 business days.